A Boston Marathon Journey

from
average runner
to amazing life

Jackie Kellner

Copyright © 2019 Jackie Kellner

All rights reserved.
No part of this book may be reproduced, scanned, or distributed in any printed or electronic form without permission.

Printed in the United States of America

ISBN: 978-1-939237-66-8

Published by Suncoast Digital Press, Inc.

Sarasota, Florida, USA

Cover photo of author: Justin Torpy Photography

Dedication

To my husband and best friend, Roy,

who always makes me laugh
and brings out the best in me.

The information provided in this book is designed to provide helpful information on the subjects discussed. This book is not meant to be used, nor should it be used, to diagnose or treat any medical condition. For diagnosis or treatment of any medical problem, consult your own physician. The publisher and author are not responsible for any specific health needs that may require medical supervision and are not liable for any damages or negative consequences from any treatment, action, application or preparation, to any person reading or following the information in this book

Contents

Foreword ix

Preface xiii

Introduction xix

1. The Early Years 1
2. The Start 7
3. Marine Corps Marathon #1 9
4. The Dark Years .13
5. Marine Corps Marathon #2 17
6. Marine Corps Marathon #3 21
7. Marine Corps Marathon #4 25
8. The Inaugural Walt Disney World Marathon 29
9. New York City Marathon #1 33
10. Walt Disney Marathon #2 39
11. Boston Marathon Replay 43
12. Time for a Change—Once Again 45
13. Roy—A New Beginning 49
14. Marine Corps Marathon #5 57

v

15. Walt Disney World Marathon #3 59
16. Key West, Florida 65
17. New York City Marathon #2. 69
18. Walt Disney World Marathon #4 73
19. Walt Disney World Marathon #5 77
20. My Florida Dream Comes True 83
21. Walt Disney World Marathon #6 87
22. Walt Disney World Marathon #7 89
23. Health 93
24. Race Day Routines. 99
25. Our Move to Melbourne 103
26. Walt Disney World Marathon #8 107
27. Boston Marathon Bombing 111
28. Walt Disney World Marathon #9 115
29. Space Coast Marathon 119
30. Sign-Up Day for the Boston Marathon 125
31. Cedar Key, Florida. 127
32. Training for Boston 131
33. Publix Florida Half Marathon 133
34. The Boston Marathon 137
35. The Year After Boston 151

36. Hurricane Matthew Comes to Call –
Twice! 155

37. Space Coast Half Marathon 159

38. The 30-Year-Old Book. 161

39. The End?. 167

Acknowledgements 171

Foreword

By Denise Piercy

Running Zone is so much more than a store that my husband, Don, and I have owned and operated for sixteen years. We are a resource center for beginners, triathletes, and anyone interested in exercise. We have taken a stand for the improvement of health and fitness in our community. In 2008, we established the Running Zone Foundation, Inc., a 501(c)(3) organization with the purpose to promote exercise and fitness and give back to our local community here in Brevard County, Florida. Today, it consists of 7 Race Series events and 6 other Foundation events. Jackie Kellner runs in these events, and knows first-hand that the wide-reaching benefits of running are personal, communal, and global.

Jackie is one of the most giving individuals I have ever met. She and her husband have hosted a water station in our Space Coast Marathon for the past 13 years. Our event has grown to over 7000 participants, which makes the support at the water/aid stations a very large task. The reviews from our participants always indicate that Jackie and Roy's station is one of the best and most enthusiastic along the course.

In addition to helping out at the Space Coast Marathon each year, Jackie volunteered to be the race director for one of our county's largest 5K road races. She was a fantastic director of that event and did a great job in raising significant funds for the non-profit organization. She introduced imaginative new ideas that year to help continue the quality and caliber that the participants expect.

Qualifying for the Boston Marathon is one of the most exciting things for a runner to accomplish. I was lucky enough to share in Jackie's joy and accomplishment when she got the exciting news that she was "in" for Boston. That feeling is almost indescribable when you finish the qualifying marathon and you know you did well.

Yes, *A Boston Marathon Journey* is a book about running, but it, too, has wide-reaching benefits to readers who are looking for an interesting story with some good tips and a whole lot of inspiration. Many new or beginner runners come into my store for advice all the time. One thing I say to every one of them is just what you can learn from this book: *We all struggle and have bad days. Don't let those days discourage you!*

A Boston Marathon Journey is not only for those aspiring to run marathons, but includes information and tips that new or average runners will find motivating, practical, and useful. Recently I was asked, "What do you think the biggest benefits are for someone to sign up for road races, even if they are 'average' runners?"

- To give them a goal to work towards; gives purpose to every day.
- Road races are very social and can be a lot of fun—this encourages you to want to do more.
- When you participate with your family, it introduces exercise as a lifestyle for children—exercise is FUN!

I am very excited to introduce to you this book, a great story of how many of us do not imagine ourselves being able to do big things in our lives, and yet somehow we do manage to achieve them.

I am always thankful for people like Jackie in our community—reading her story helps us to realize that we all have such different backgrounds and paths that bring us to together as a community, and more specifically, a running family.

I hope you enjoy her story and feel confident you will be inspired by it as well.

        Denise Piercy
        Co-owner, Running Zone
        Melbourne, Florida

        Co-Founder,
        Running Zone Foundation, Inc.,
        Non-profit established to promote fitness and benefit local charities

Preface

"Life is either one daring adventure, or nothing."
—Helen Keller

April 18, 2016–Hopkinton, Massachusetts

It's almost 10:30 a.m. My start time for the Boston Marathon is 11:15 a.m. and my group (Wave 4) has been called to the start. By this time of day I am normally at the finish line of a marathon, having started around 6:00 a.m. I am looking around, and trying to figure out how I got here. This does not feel real. It must be a dream.

This is my 18th and probably the last marathon I will run. I am 67 years old.

It is a beautiful morning here, nothing like the stories I'd heard from friends who ran the Boston Marathon. They spoke of cold temperatures, maybe with rain or high winds. Today the temperature is in the low 60s with sun and not much of a breeze. This is more like Florida weather where I now live and train year-round.

"God, I hope I can do this." Walking to the start, I have to keep telling myself, "You can *do this!" Luckily, I am a positive person. My journey has been long and sometimes bumpy to get to this point and I* will *finish this marathon. Roy, my wonderful husband and biggest supporter, is waiting for me at the finish.*

I look at the houses as I walk to the start and think about what a nice town Hopkinton is. I have always liked small towns. While standing at the start of the race I notice a small church to my left. I look at the church and thank God in advance that I am having a good race but most of all a safe run. I don't want to trip and fall down. I notice all of the security – men on top of the buildings with rifles. I am not afraid. I feel very secure.

How did I get to the Boston Marathon? It was never on my bucket list. I am just an average runner. I ran the Marine Corps Marathon five times, Disney in Orlando nine times, New York City twice and the Space Coast Marathon once. I had decent finish times but not Joan Samuelson finish times. I am short at five feet, two inches and I weigh 117 pounds. I do not have long, thin legs. My stride is short. And I am a sixty-seven-year-old grandmother. Still, I love to run and train.

I have a special blessing that I say just before I start a training run or a race and I say it now, "Thank You God for this beautiful Massachusetts morning. Thank You that I am having a good and safe run. I am very grateful."

The gun goes off for the start. I start the timer on my running watch as I cross the start mat. I begin the mantra which I will say a million times over the next 26.2 miles: "I am blessed, thank You."

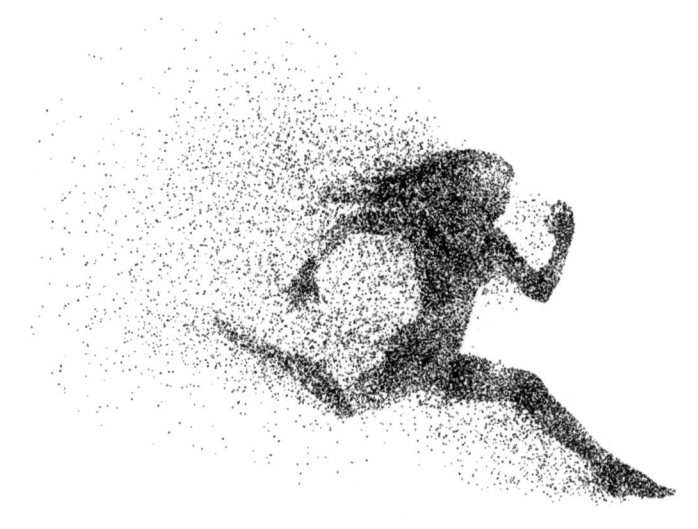

> "Life isn't about finding yourself.
> Life is about creating yourself."
>
> —George Bernard Shaw

I admit to knowing the lyrics to most all Jimmy Buffett songs. I'm thinking of when he wrote that just the act of getting something down on paper can help one make sense of it. Writing a book has been a dream of mine since the sixth grade, but I never knew what to write about, until now. Desire combined with purpose, finally, as I endeavored to make sense of how I came to qualify for and run the Boston Marathon at the age of 67.

The Boston Marathon was never on my bucket list, although prior to my Boston run in 2016 I had completed seventeen marathons. After I completed a marathon under my qualifying time, I applied for Boston, was accepted, and my fate was sealed.

This book is an attempt to try and figure out how and why this happened. I always thought of myself as just an average runner, but completing the Boston Marathon meant I was average no longer. Out of the entire U.S. population, only 0.5% have ever run 26.2 miles, or 42 kilometers, a distance known as a "marathon." Out of all American runners, 45% have run a marathon. Out of that group, just 10.4% have qualified for Boston. The Boston Marathon is unlike other marathons, which is part of its appeal and prestige. You can't just sign up whenever you wish. You need a qualifying time (based on your age and gender) from another marathon, and that qualifying time has to have been run with a set date range on a certain type of course. Preference is given to those who have submitted the fastest qualifying times. What were the odds of me finding myself among thousands of runners in Boston on Patriot's Day when I had only dreamed of such an opportunity, being the average runner I knew myself to me?

Just get started—dreams do come true!

As you read my story, I want to encourage both women and men who consider themselves average, like I did, to embrace the fact that you can still accomplish amazing things. We all can't be elite runners, but we can accomplish more than we first realize.

This is not simply a book to encourage you to run. It is to encourage you to live. Clearly, to live your life to the fullest, good health is a requirement. There are many forms of exercise and you should choose the one that best suits you. I am an example of someone who discovered running in my 30s and kept with it. I share my running story with people I meet, especially people over the age of 30. It is never too late to start taking care of your body and start an exercise program. I learned that firsthand. Thankfully, I came to understand that

God gave me this body and it is my responsibility to take care of it.

As I look back through my running logs, which date back to 1983, I can see that as each year passes I continue to make running my passion and priority and I continue to get healthier every year. There were some dark and challenging years from time to time, but I got through them. I believe running helped to keep me going. No, I *know* it did. I had at least one positive something to look forward to each morning to start my day. Running gave me courage and confidence and I learned that I could depend on and trust running.

Now, nearly four decades after discovering running, I still run five days a week, 25 miles or more every week. I have nine grandchildren, and I still wear a two-piece swimsuit when I go to the beach!

Introduction

> "I don't know how to do this
> but something inside me does."
> —Paul Williams

I heard this quote just as I started writing my book and it was perfect. I wrote it on a piece of paper and taped it to my desk so I would see it when I sat down to work. I said this so many times to myself it has become a part of me. I probably say it in my sleep.

To meet any challenge, it is important to find quotes, stories, and/or personal heroes to inspire you.

One of the extra bedrooms in our home is my running room. There is so much history and so many great memories in that room. On one wall are all of the finisher medals from my half marathons and marathons—all except for my first, the 1984 Marine Corps Marathon, because there were no finisher medals that year, only t-shirts. My awards are displayed on the bookcase, all four walls, desk, and futon (the stuffed animals I won at the Brevard Zoo 2-Mile Race), and even on the floor.

I've had a subscription to *Runner's World* magazine since they merged with *The Runner* and I kept every issue for over 25 years. Those magazines kept stacking up and went with me each time I moved. I finally recycled all but a few special issues which now have a perfect home in my running room.

Among these treasures are the May 1981 Silver Anniversary Collector's issue of *Runner's World* with Frank Shorter on the cover, and *The Runner* September 1981 issue with Gayle Barron on the cover. I have copies of the October 1984 issue of *The Runner* and the October 1984 *Runner's World*, both of which featured Joan Benoit on the cover after she finished first in the marathon at the Summer Olympics in Los Angeles, California. I met Joan some years later at Running Zone running store in Melbourne, Florida, and she autographed both copies. She was very surprised I still had both copies of the magazines. I will always remember the smile she gave me. Joan is my hero, maybe because she is five feet, two inches tall, just like me.

I have the farewell issue of *The Runner* (April 1987). I also kept the *Runner's World* July 2013 issue after the Boston bombing. I read this issue twice and cried both times.

Also stacked on the bookcase are running logs dating back to the 1983 *Complete Runner's Day-by-Day Log and Calendar* by James Fixx. I had read two of his books and decided to try his running log. It was a good choice. This not only tracks my miles and routes, it has kept me motivated year-to-year. It is empowering to look at all you have accomplished and at all your progress.

> Start using a day-to-day running log.
> Down the road, you will be so glad you did.

On January first, I go through the log book month by month and write down the races I plan to run. Looking back, I have found a lot of very useful notations in these logs. The first few years I wrote very little information, mostly my mileage and very few personal details. The past 25 years have much more detail. The only years I did not purchase a log were 1986, 1989, and 1990. These were some of my darker years.

Before I used running logs, I started a scrapbook. This was right after my very first race, The Best Running & Fitness Day Festival and 12K on October 9, 1982, at Washington D.C.'s West Potomac Park. This scrapbook is 12" x 14", and while I never thought I would run enough races to fill it up, I did. I figured that I'd be too old to run after the age of 40. Was I ever wrong! The scrapbook is full of my race bibs, pictures, race flyers, and a few newspaper articles about the races I ran.

The first race I remember placing in my age group was the Alexandria Autumn 10K on October 14, 1984, when I finished 2nd place in my age group of women 35-39. My finish time was 46:54. I did not run a race in 1986. I ran one race in 1989 and two races in 1990. Those were some of my dark years. Also, there were fewer races put on during those years as compared to the vast opportunities we have today.

Recently friends have asked how many races I have run through the years. As I went through my scrapbook and running logs, I discovered I have run 18 marathons and 32 half marathons, and a total number of 334 other races of different distances, as of the end of 2017.

This is not a very large number compared to some runners I know who have run *over a thousand races*. I am not the type of runner who runs a race every weekend. I just want to continue to run and race and not get injured or burned out.

I have had many dreams come true in the past 20-something years, some which you'll read about on the following pages.

Writing a book to share my running journey with you is also a dream come true. I sincerely hope you will discover and follow your own dreams that transport you from "average" to "amazing." So here I go. Like my husband always tells me when I leave for a training run or before I start a race, "Run fast!"

1

The Early Years

*Never give up on your dream.
Just because it may not happen right away
doesn't mean it never will.*

The first time I thought about writing a book, I was in the sixth grade. Sitting in our living room with my sister and a girlfriend doing our homework, I had just started writing a story when my mother came home from work. I announced to her that I was writing a book. "That's nice." She never said another word or asked about why I wanted to write a book. Well, that was that. I tossed the paper and discarded the idea.

I did not grow up in a happy home full of inspiration, as I imagine would be idyllic. In fact, there was so much *missing*—encouragement, aspirational thoughts, discussion of why accomplishments were meaningful and that the future was worth working toward, perhaps college…As do many children in dysfunctional homes, I found a way to escape and mine was by reading books. One reason I learned to read at an early age was that my pleas to be read to fell on deaf ears. But what a wonderful thing it was to be able to read, to transport myself into stories any time I wanted. Yes, I had hoped for a bit of encouragement when I shared my dream of writing a book; I was to learn later in life that I had to be my own champion.

I was never drawn to sports and remember myself as a chubby little girl growing up in the early 1950s in Atlanta, Georgia. I was required to participate in outside activities in grammar school, went through two years of dance lessons, and took the gym classes that high school dictated. My mother and grandmother were constantly admonishing me to not get dirty, so I never wanted to get rumpled, sweaty, or, heaven forbid, mess up my hair. All of that changed (completely!) once I started running.

> *"I am not athletic"*
> *can change to*
> *"I love physical activity"*
> *at any point in life!*

My mother was a very controlling person. I grew up thinking that was normal, and I ended up marrying one controlling man, and then another. My first husband was also physically abusive. I finally left but got into a second marriage that was probably worse than the first. I tried changing both husbands but that did not work. I learned that I had to change myself and finally say no to the physical and mental abuse I had suffered. I made a healthy decision to stay away from my mother for many years. Her criticism and anger were toxic to me as a child, and carried through to adulthood....as long as I put up with it. I went to visit her shortly after my second marriage. Because of running, I was very fit and had lost a lot of weight but she could not say I looked great. She only said, "Be careful that you don't gain all of that weight back." This felt so much like when she used to actually slap my face. Once I finally said to myself, *no more abuse*, it meant

NO MORE to anyone in my life: husband, mother, friends, anyone—past, present, or future.

I was getting stronger on the inside and knew something had to change. That little voice inside of me was screaming for my attention, and I was beginning to listen. It was running that gave me the confidence and the courage to walk out on husband number one and husband number two, and to become my own "abuse-free zone."

My parents divorced when I was around eight years old. My mother hated my daddy and reminded me of that almost every day. I remember when he moved out of our house, carrying a suitcase and saying he would not be back. My grandmother told me years later that I cried so hard she thought I would cry my eyes out. I felt very empty on the inside for years. To this day I think I reminded my mother too much of my daddy, so she did not like me much either.

My daddy had visitation, but after a few years that fell apart. He remarried and started another family. I did get back in touch with him years later and I was able to spend an afternoon with him before he died. I will always be grateful for that afternoon. We did a lot of talking and I was able to tell him that I loved him.

I also discovered that he had my original birth certificate. I had asked my mother for this several times over the years, and she only said she did not have it, not that my father probably did. He said it was the one thing he wanted and took it before he left. He gave it to me and I still have it.

I will not go into much detail but after my parents divorced, one of my mother's boyfriends sexually abused me and my sister. I was only in 6th grade. I did not tell my mother because I felt I had done something wrong and that she would beat me if she knew. But my sister told my grandmother. Our grandmother told our daddy and he took us to the police station to have a report written.

My mother and her boyfriend told us to say it never happened. They bribed us with a milkshake and Silly Putty, and warned us with silent but deadly glares. Of course, we obeyed her so we would not get the belt. Mother never asked if the abuse happened. She never took us to the doctor. She just acted like our dad had made it all up. I was an adult before I had the courage to bring the subject up to her. She said it was my fault.

During my years of therapy I finally had the courage to discuss the abuse with someone. I told the therapist that for years my mother denied that the abuse happened. The therapist suggested that if my mother had admitted the abuse had happened she would be admitting that she was not perfect. Good point.

In my attempts to heal my childhood wounds, I tried talking to her a few times through the years, but that did not work. She died from cancer over 23 years ago. Through years of reading self-help books, and then from running, I eventually learned to be positive and try to make something of myself. I thank each of the writers whose books I read and continue to read to this day.

I love that being older means I can look back on my darker years and see them very differently. I have learned the power of forgiveness. I have learned to look for and embrace the lessons from life and I can see purpose in those difficult years. I can see now that I was growing and learning, and that my mistakes were helping me do that. Of course, I did not realize it at the time. I just felt lost and stuck.

I was doing all sorts of things to try and figure out if my future would be any better, almost as if it was already scripted. I was reading books about crystals and crystal healing. I consulted a man who could tell you about your past lives and give some insight into the future. I had my palm read, and at least three different people told me I would be married three times and have four children. Now wait a minute...I was already in my second marriage. I did not want to be a two-time loser. And three more children? No way. It started to occur to me that there was no glimpsing some set-in-stone future, that it really was up to me to design and make a life for myself, one that matched my deepest desires.

From a very early age I wanted to have a baby, especially a boy—maybe because my parents divorced when I was young and I did not see much of my father. I had one sister but no brothers. I was a little boy-crazy.

My first husband was in the Air Force. A few months before our baby was born in 1968, my husband received orders to be stationed in Myrtle Beach, South Carolina. A couple of months after moving to Myrtle Beach we were assigned base housing. Pink or blue? The second bedroom was always already painted either pink or blue, and you never knew which you would get. Our second bedroom was blue, and I sure hoped that meant we would have a boy. My son Johnny was born November 21...my first genuine and lasting dream-come-true.

My little boy was so special to me and I was happy taking care of him. An inner voice told me one child would be enough for me, so at age 29, I decided on a procedure called tubal ligation; I did not just want the tubes tied, I wanted them clipped and burned. I have never regretted that decision.

Today I am married for the third time and my husband gave me three wonderful stepsons. Yes, it turns out I'm twice divorced and have four children. BUT, I am absolutely not a loser, nor do I have my palms read any longer. I've created a beautiful, active life with a loving husband and fantastic friends here in Florida, and I have finally found the peace and happiness that were inside me all along.

As a child growing up, I thought 30 was old. Was I ever wrong. As Diana Nyad said, "Age doesn't matter when you are chasing a dream."

> We are capable of much more than we realize.
> What might you be capable of,
> if you simply took the first step?

I have learned that people are capable of much more than they realize, although it took some time. I needed to learn to get over my fears and insecurities in order to keep moving forward. I could come across as a very confident, strong person, but that was only on the outside. There was so much inside of me that I could not share. I just pushed it all down deeper and deeper through the years. I am so grateful that I found myself through running. With each planted foot, I was gaining strength in my core being. With each lifted foot, I was leaving my insecurities and negative energy from the past behind on the pavement.

2

The Start

Have the courage to try something new.

A few years earlier in 1979, still living in Georgia, a couple of my co-workers started running during the lunch hour after the Christmas holidays. They said it was the quickest way to take off the extra holiday weight. I remembered myself as a chubby child, and I normally carried ten to twenty pounds of extra weight that I was never happy with. I had tried every type of fad diet through the years. I would lose a few pounds then gain it back every time. Now I had the answer to keeping the extra weight off and I was hooked. I had finally found the secret, or so I thought at the time.

I moved from Georgia with my first husband and 11-year-old son to Alexandria, Virginia. One of my new co-workers, Becky, was a runner and she talked about racing and running a marathon. She told me she ran 10 miles on Saturdays and I just did not believe that was possible for me, or that anyone other than an Olympian could ever run 26 miles.

Then I started thinking. *Would'nt it be amazing if I could run a marathon?* Becky suggested I try a few shorter races first, and to increase my weekly efforts. I had never trained for or run a race. There was a running trail near my house that I could walk to, so I started putting in a few miles just a couple of days a week.

I signed up for my first race, The Best Running & Fitness Day Festival and 12K, which was held on October 9, 1982. I thought I would die a mile before the finish but the friend I was running with encouraged me to keep going. My official finish time was 1:06:25. This was a few years before chip timing and I did not have a running watch in order to time myself.

Finishing that race gave me a real boost and I began to run around my neighborhood before going to work each morning. I also joined my first health club, the Skyline Fitness Center, and I would go there after work for exercise classes and sometimes do another run outside or on the indoor track.

A few months after moving to Virginia, I'd finally had enough of my husband's abuse. I moved out of the house we were renting and we started divorce proceedings. He was never supportive of my running, but I was now free to do the things I wanted—finally free of fear, or so I thought.

3

Marine Corps Marathon #1
November 4, 1984 – Washington, D.C.

There is nothing like a first marathon. You will question your good sense many times.

On an early Sunday morning on August 5, 1984, I sat down to watch the summer Olympics taking place in Los Angeles, California. This was the first Olympics in which there was finally a women's marathon. Joan Benoit, my hero, was running for the United States. I had just signed up for my first marathon and I needed to see her win. Joan took off quickly, considering the heat. The announcer commented that she would not last and would fade because of going out this fast. She even skipped the first water station.

Joan became the first woman to win the marathon in the Olympics. I will never forget the look on her face and her smile, full of pride and happiness with her accomplishment, as she crossed the finish line. I wanted that feeling. Now I was pumped, determined, and full of confidence for my first marathon.

I was at Skyline on Friday evening before the Marine Corps Marathon, taking a short run on the indoor track. After my run I was talking to a couple of guys about the marathon. One of the guys asked what I thought my finish time would be and I said under four hours. He just laughed and said, "No one finishes a first marathon in under four hours."

The race started at 9:00 a.m. and I was ready. I had not followed a training plan or run with a group during training, just read a book or two and a couple of magazines. I was totally naïve but confident. Training for the marathon was not so technical in those days, at least not what I knew of it.

The weather was really nice, which for me meant no rain and above 32 degrees. According to my running log I never felt bad during the race. The course for this marathon is really beautiful. You can see a lot more of Washington D.C. by foot rather than by car. There was much cheering from the spectators along the course, making me feel like an elite runner.

My plan for running the marathon was to not take a walk break until Mile 20 and to be at Mile 20 within three hours. I made it to Mile 20 in 2:46. I had a finish time for a 10K of 45:57, so I knew I would have almost an hour to finish the last 6.2 miles of the marathon, and that I could take some walk breaks if I felt I needed them.

The last six miles were the hardest, but running up that last hill to the finish, I felt fantastic. I was very happy with my time and the marathon. My plan—having no plan—really worked.

The one problem I experienced after I crossed the finish line was that I did not know about eating and drinking plenty of water after the race. There was plenty of food at the finish, but I was too pumped to eat. I went home, opened a bottle of champagne, and called a couple of friends. Then I decided to take a shower. That's when the champagne hit me, and I almost passed out. I made it to my bed and lay there for a couple of hours before I got up to eat. Lesson learned.

On Monday after work I went back to the club and the same guy asked me about my finish time. I said 3:59:02. He never discussed finish times with me again. But that was fine because I had decided this was my first *and* last marathon. There was no reason to go through this training again. After running 26.2 miles, my confidence was at an all-time high. I now felt I could accomplish anything I put my mind to. That feeling did not last very long.

4

The Dark Years

A lot can be learned about yourself during hard times.

The year after my first marathon was not a happy one. I was now in my second marriage, which had turned out to be much worse than the first. We had fun when we first met but things changed very quickly. We lived on the seventeenth floor of a high-rise apartment building with a great view in Alexandria, Virginia, and I hated it.

While I was unhappy most days, I don't think I was clinically depressed. I didn't have a problem getting up each morning. I had a job at a personnel agency that I really loved and I continued to go to the Skyline Fitness Center each day after work. But something was missing from my life.

I took some time off from running after hearing that it was good to let the body heal after a marathon, but that just made me feel worse. My motivation was very low. As my thirty-sixth birthday approached on December 10, there were no celebrations planned.

There are few notes written in my logs from the years 1984 to early 1991. I do complain about being tired a lot. I continued to enjoy my job with the personnel agency, as I was helping people find jobs and that was very rewarding. I was still running and exercising, but I had no interest in racing. I seemed to be happy during the day but miserable when at home, still in that very unhealthy second marriage.

In my 1985 running log, I listed three goals on the first page: run a total of 2,500 miles, break 45 minutes in a 10K, and complete the Marine Corps Marathon in 3:20. I cannot say that I accomplished any of those goals. I ran one 10K but did not write down my finish time. I did not track my mileage for the year. I have very few notes past March.

I did not purchase a log in 1986. In the 1987 log, I listed no goals for the year, and I wrote very little about my personal life. I must have wanted to forget as much as possible about those years living in Virginia. I may have been concerned that someone would read my logs one day or just didn't want to put that misery down on paper. I can only see a dark tunnel when I think back on those years.

One bright spot was a new health club, The Center Club, which opened in May right next door to the building where I lived and only one mile from my office. I took exercise classes, worked out on the equipment, and ran on the indoor track. I ran a total of 741 miles for the year but did not compete in any road races.

The 1988 log looks very similar to 1987. I continued going to The Center Club almost daily after work, and I ran a total of 605 miles for the year.

The next log was in 1991. There were no goals listed. My mileage increased to 1,452 for the year but my personal life took a turn. After about eight years of being so unhappy in the second marriage, I realized I was drinking too much. In

January I decided to stop drinking alcohol, start running again each day, and move into the second bedroom while I took six months to figure out what I needed to do.

The country was in a recession and I was not making much money. Moving out and trying to make it on my own would not be easy, but anything would be better than my current situation. I had a part-time job in a book store and was still working at the personnel agency.

"Strength does not come from winning. Your struggles develop your strengths. When you go through hardships and decide not to surrender, that is strength." —Arnold Schwarzenegger

What helped me the most to get through this miserable phase was running and exercise. After being beaten down for so many years, I needed to work on my confidence and courage. Although I was still not running as much as I had when I trained for the Marine Corps Marathon, my mileage was starting to pick up and I was feeling much better.

I was getting zero support and motivation from home and even counseling was not helping to keep the marriage together. Husband number two did not feel he needed to change one bit. After the six-month period, I moved out on June 20, 1991. Thank God we did not have children. Johnny was 23 at the time and living in College Station, Texas, as a student at Texas A&M University.

During this time one of my good friends committed suicide. We had worked at the same personnel agency for a time and sat in the same office, so we talked a lot. My second husband didn't like her, so after she moved on from the agency we hadn't seen each other for several months. I missed her and invited her to meet me for lunch. I had just read a book that I really liked and planned to loan it to her. She killed herself the night before we were to meet. I knew she had problems, but I never saw that coming. I will never forget her. I still think of her to this day and what a waste it has been to lose her. In some ways, it made me more determined to get myself over and out of of my darker days, sooner than later.

5

Marine Corps Marathon #2
November 3, 1991 – Washington, D.C.

Never say "never again."

I said I was finished after the first one, but there I was, seven years later, lined up for the start.

My son was now in the Navy ROTC program at Texas A&M and he and his friends were planning to be inducted into the Marine Corps as officers after graduation. He called me at the end of June and said he and some buddies were planning to run the Marine Corps Marathon and wanted to know if I would also run.

I had not run or raced much those past seven years, though in 1990 I did finally run a couple of 10Ks again. I was trying to get motivated to get back to long-distance running, and I figured signing up for the Marine Corps Marathon and seeing my son would be just the impetus I needed.

I had been in a dark place for most of the past seven years and was now into my second divorce. I had moved out of the high-rise building and into my own apartment—on the first floor. The recession continued and the job that I loved and was very successful in for the last seven years was no more.

There were very few available jobs out there and I needed training for a new career.

Still, my life seemed to be going much better. I was more motivated, and looked forward to running each day. I met a new guy who lived in Annapolis, Maryland. There was nothing for me in Virginia, so I was considering moving to Annapolis. As it turned out, it was the best move I ever made.

My training for the marathon went very well and I had a great race, not stopping for a walk break until Mile 25. I finished strong and felt great, and my new boyfriend and his youngest daughter met me at the finish.

As I look back, I am surprised I finished the first couple of marathons as well as I did without a coach, a training plan, or 20-mile training runs. I was running 40- to 60-miles per week, but my long runs were never longer than 14 miles.

At the last minute my son decided not to come to Alexandria and run the marathon, though his buddies did. After his buddies returned to College Station, Texas, he told me his buddies were talking about their finish times, which were around 4:15, 4:25, and 4:45. They asked Johnny about my finish time and he said 3:55:41. He was so proud and the guys, of course, were very surprised. How could a woman my age have a faster finish time than any of these guys who were training to be tough Marines?

By the spring of 1992, I had moved to Annapolis, Maryland, into my boyfriend's house. I had joined the Annapolis Striders Running Club and my running and racing were really taking off. Joining a running club made such a difference. I made some new running friends and, after a few more years, I would start to join them for long runs on Saturday mornings. At that time, though, I just could not get myself up early on Saturday to run a 10 mile training run after working all week. I was running the club's series races and a few other local races. During the week I would run from the house to the Annapolis City Dock and back. My confidence was up those days.

6

Marine Corps Marathon #3
October 25, 1992 – Washington, D.C.

Never give up.
We never know what tomorrow will bring.

As the year went on, things got harder. Leading up to the marathon I was tired, depressed and just not happy. I was looking for a job but there was very little to choose from, and I was worried about money. I would have taken just about anything at this point.

I entered my running times and miles in my running log but said very little about looking forward to the marathon. I do see one note from the Friday before the event that I was getting excited.

Something was still missing from my life. I was trying to find some happiness, looking for something, anything, outside of myself to make me happy. I had not yet learned that happiness starts from within.

There *were* two very happy occasions that year. In May I flew to College Station to see Johnny's graduation from Texas A&M, and his commencement ceremony into the Marine Corps the next day. I was back in College Station again for Johnny and his bride, Gina's military wedding on August 8th. Over the years they have given me three amazing grandchildren, two boys and a girl. All three have turned out to be very smart and athletic. They have made their parents, and their grandmother, very proud.

The situation with my boyfriend went down pretty quickly after I moved in, but I stayed with him for three years. I thought I could make things better. We seemed to argue a lot. He was not a physically violent person, just selfish and self-centered. He had been married twice and had three children. The two oldest were grown and he had a 12-year-old daughter. He was not very nice to his children or his mother. Seems like I would have realized that was a big red flag.

I found a couple of jobs in the summer but neither lasted too long. Between that and the arguing with my boyfriend, I felt stuck again. Finally, in September, I started a full-time job with a chiropractor. At first I assisted with the physical therapy before learning medical billing. I enjoyed working with the doctor and the patients. I was learning so much about how the body works and I was getting very interested in health.

I continued to work for doctors in several different fields for another twenty years until I no longer need to work. I learned medical billing and collections and this also gave me the opportunity to help patients with their balances.

I finished my third marathon in 4:35:03. The weather was beautiful but with wind blowing at 25 miles per hour. Everyone was complaining about the wind. I ran eight-minute miles the first seven miles, then I just ran out of energy. I took a lot of walk breaks the last seven miles and I was not happy with my time.

I still had no training plan or schedule except to run every day, and my long runs on the weekend were just over 14 miles—even when I was training for the marathon. I was still getting in 40-60 miles every week, mainly because I ran just about every day.

It is very sad to read back through my running logs and see how unhappy I was during those years. The chiropractor I worked for was trying to help with my weight and lack of energy, though I may have been tired because I ran every morning and was on my feet all day at work in a busy practice. When the office closed to patients for an hour each day at lunchtime, I would stay there and eat, then lay on a treatment table and rest for a while.

Yet there is a reason I made it through so many dark years without just giving up. Things would change for me, but it would take another three years.

7

Marine Corps Marathon #4
October 24, 1993 – Washington, D.C.

Writing down personal and running goals can keep you motivated and committed.

My fourth Marine Corps Marathon was just before my forty-fifth birthday. At first I couldn't figure out why I'd signed up for this one, then I remembered—it was to honor my son, now an officer in the Marine Corps. Johnny and Gina were stationed in California, and he called two weeks before the marathon to let me know I was going to be a grandmother for the first time.

I even wore a special shirt for this and the two previous Marine Corps Marathons. On the front it says, "My son is a U.S. Marine," and to the back I added, "You are following the mom of Lt. John Skinner USMC." I got more than a few comments during the race. I still have this shirt hanging in my closet.

I was still a member of the Annapolis Striders Running Club and, according to my running log, my weekly mileage had picked up, so I assume my motivation must have been up as well. I was running 30-, 40- and 50-mile weeks. I was working a four-day work week at the chiropractor's office with Fridays off so that's when I did my long runs. I was running seven days a week and I took very few rest days. I hadn't learned yet that rest days are important to let the body heal.

I started a 15-week training program for the marathon on July 15 and my goal was to finish under four hours, though I am not clear where this plan came from. This meant I was more focused on the long runs and on getting in my shorter runs each day. I hadn't started to train with the Annapolis Striders on Saturdays; I was only running local races with them.

I can see in my log that my long runs did pick up and I put in two 18-mile training runs before the marathon, along with the Annapolis 10 Mile Run on August 29 (in 1:29:58) and the 13th Annual Metric (16.10 miles) Marathon (in 2:24:39).

I was also now writing down my running and personal goals for the year. I must have been in a better place those days. At least I was more focused and planning for my future, one year at a time. My running goals were mainly races I planned to run that year: Bay Bridge, Annapolis 10 Mile Race, Marine Corps Marathon, and the Cherry Blossom 10 Mile Race in D.C. My personal goals were pretty basic: lose weight, stay in the best of health, and get my life together.

On the morning of the Marine Corps Marathon, the weather was just about perfect, with clear blue skies and a very light breeze. I felt great until about Mile 18, when I tripped and went down on the 14th Street bridge. I felt as if my feet just stopped and the top of my body kept going forward, and I went down.

Two guys pulled me up very quickly and we just kept running. I was only down for a second. One guy stayed with me until he was sure I was okay. Nothing was broken except my pride.

Everything happened too fast for me to stop and think about the reason I fell. I would try to figure it out after the finish.

My Annapolis boyfriend had promised me a special present if I finished under four hours, but I never found out what that present would have been. My finish time was 4:08:43, which was not bad. I would have finished under four hours had I not fallen. It usually takes me a few minutes to catch my breath and get back into rhythm after a fall. The day after the marathon, my legs were a little more sore as compared to the previous three marathons. I went outside for walks each day for some exercise. I don't see any notes in my running log that I was doing much stretching those days. By Thursday I was starting to feel normal again and I started running again the following Sunday. I seemed to heal very quickly.

I had signed up for the inaugural Walt Disney Marathon in January 1994, so I couldn't waste too much time before getting back into training. I hoped I had made the right decision to run two marathons so close together. But it was Disney, after all, so I told myself I would crawl to the finish if that's what it took.

I ran over 2,000 miles in 1993 but I was still not happy in my personal life. The only constant in my life was running; it was the only thing I really seemed to look forward to each day.

8

The Inaugural Walt Disney World Marathon
January 16, 1994 – Orlando, Florida

You do not have to compete against anyone else, but always challenge yourself to do your best.

I flew from Annapolis to Orlando to run the inaugural Walt Disney World Marathon. When I saw the advertisement in *Runner's World* magazine about this marathon I *had* to sign up. I grew up with the Mickey Mouse Club so there was no way I would be missing out on this one. I had only been to Disney World in Orlando once before.

My training had gone really well, and I was happy to be there. I hadn't done long runs on the weekends but I did a few on Wednesdays. I was not following a training plan, just running almost every day with very few days off. One of my long runs was the Cold Turkey 20K on November 28, 1993, where I placed third in the women's 40-49 division with a time of 1:46:14. I hadn't placed very often in my age group, so I was very happy.

Arriving on Friday, I checked into the Beach Resort Hotel, a Disney property. From there I could take a Disney bus to any place I needed to go within the property as well as to the start of the marathon Sunday morning. I went to the Expo to check out the exhibits and pick up my race packet. I still have the long-sleeve race t-shirt that came with that packet.

> *Traveling alone has its rewards, so don't let fear of it stop you from following your dream.*

I had a great time on my own. It was freeing to only have myself to listen to about what I wanted to see or eat or experience, at any given time. I took a boat ride to Fort Wilderness for a short run on Friday afternoon and again on Saturday morning. It was so beautiful there. The grass was green, and all of the hibiscuses were in bloom. When I left Annapolis on Friday, the temperature was in the 30s with ice on the streets.

On race day the temperature was 51 degrees at the 6:00 a.m. start at Epcot. The sun came up about an hour after the race started. My goal was to run under four hours but by Mile 10, I realized that would not happen. The beginning of the race had been so tight with the other runners I couldn't get up enough speed. All of the runners started the race at the same time and I had to slow down too much on the turns until we were out on the roads that connect the parks.

My second goal was to run the entire course without a walk break, which was challenging since the Disney parks are so beautiful, especially with the early start. We started and finished at Epcot, running through the Magic Kingdom, Blizzard Beach, and Disney MGM Studios. I wanted to stop and take it all in, but I just kept running. Any time I felt like taking a walk break, my ego kept me going.

That first Disney marathon had very few spectators. I believe we only had the Disney characters, volunteers, and park staff. Over time this has changed. The park is now open earlier on race days so there are lots of spectators who cheer very loudly for the runners. Spectators can make a big difference.

I did run the entire 26.2 miles without a walk break, just grabbing water and Gatorade as needed. My finish time was 4:08:37 and I finished 45 out of 183 women in my age group of 45-49, so a little above average. I decided then that I would run the first five Disney Marathons. I don't know where I came up with that number. Looks like I have stopped telling myself that this will be my "last" marathon. I feel I can now run marathons forever.

Each year there have been good improvements to the Disney course and the marathon has become much more crowded with runners. The early days of everyone starting at the same time are over; the runners now start in waves and according to their estimated finish time.

After the race I took the bus back to the hotel, showered, packed, and headed to the airport. I was starting a new job the next day. I had very little soreness in my legs and no blisters on my feet. Arriving in Maryland, I was welcomed with snow and ice everywhere. This was probably the best reason to keep running the Disney Marathon each January—at least I could escape the northeast weather for a few days.

9

New York City Marathon #1
November 4, 1994

Train on hills. You will learn to love it.

After one last treatment from my chiropractor, I took the train from Annapolis to Penn Station and walked to the Novotel Hotel, which was also close to Central Park. It was daylight as I exited the train and made my way to the street, walking out into New York City for the first time in my life. This is a moment I will never forget. I enjoyed all the scenes of Times Square, especially the naked cowboy playing the guitar! I'm sure I looked like a tourist, but no one bothered me. I guess I looked like all of the other runners who had come to be part of the 25th anniversary of the New York City Marathon.

I signed up for this race on May 23, 1994, though I don't remember why. In those days you had to request that an application be mailed to you, then fill it out and return it along with your check. I was so happy to be accepted! I had never been to New York and now I would be going by myself. I was very excited, and not at all afraid about going alone. Running was giving me much needed self-confidence and courage.

On July 23, I finally decided to check out the Saturday morning group run with the Annapolis Striders Running Club, which started at 7:00 a.m. on Route 450. It was great! Most of the runners were training for the Marine Corps Marathon. I hadn't met anyone who was training for New York, but it was only a few weeks after the Marine Corps so I could just run their schedule. Water was put out for the group every two miles along with peppermint candies.

Our first training run was 10 miles. I was told that when you start marathon training, if you could not run 10 miles the first day of training then you are not ready. I was now training for marathons as I should. According to my log we ran *20* miles on September 24—I must have survived.

Route 450 has some major hills, so those Saturday morning runs taught me a lot about how to run inclines. I learned very soon that I actually enjoy running hills—it uses the muscles in the back of the legs and gives the muscles in the front of the legs a little rest.

The Saturday morning group was known as Moore's Marines, after our coach who was retired Marine Corps LTC Ben Moore. We did not have a written training plan. This was before the days when everyone had email. Ben simply let us know our distance each Saturday just before the start of the training run.

I started having low back issues in September and I did all of my training for New York through this pain. I was determined to run this marathon—especially because I had paid the fee and made hotel reservations.

I was working for a chiropractor at the time. I felt I was getting good care, but we could not figure out what was going on with my low back. A notation in my running log states *pinched nerve*. I had an X-ray but it didn't show anything serious. Once I was able to get out of bed in the mornings, the pain would pretty much subside, but bending forward to get into my running shoes was another issue. I would be in tears until I tied my shoes and could stand up.

I arrived in New York City on Friday, November 4. After checking into the hotel I went to the Expo to pick up my race packet, where I was thrilled to meet Bill Rogers for the first time. I met Bill at the Expo but, according to the notes in my running log, I did not have any additional detail. He was probably at one of the Expo booths and we just said hello to one another. At the time I did not have anything for him to autograph. I walked around for a little while but did not attend any seminars.

The next morning I went for a run in Central Park. Everyone was very friendly. This was my first trip to Central Park but would not be my last. I had always heard so much about Central Park and now there I was. I believe the park was closed to traffic on the weekends, so people were running, walking, riding bikes, and skating on the streets in the park without any worry about cars, buses, or trucks.

After going to the Expo again on Saturday I was walking on the sidewalk and could not believe I ran into Linda, another runner from the Annapolis Striders. We did not know each other would be running the New York City Marathon since she didn't run with the group on Saturdays. It turned out she had run New York many times.

On Sunday, Marathon morning, I was up very early. It was still dark outside. The buses left for Staten Island around 6:30 a.m. for the 11:00 a.m. start time. Since Linda and I were not staying at the same hotel, we decided to meet outside my hotel to ride the bus together and so Linda could show me the ropes. There was very little to do during the four-hour wait. There were a couple of weddings and some other entertainment to watch, but we did not want to spend much time walking and standing. Water, coffee and snacks were provided for the runners as we waited. It was nice to hang out with someone I knew who also happened to know just what to do on race morning.

Finally, it was time to begin walking to the start area, located just before we would run up the Verrazano-Narrows Bridge. Linda and I were very close to the start. During those days we were not required to line up according to our estimated finish time. We could see the elite female runners very close to where we were standing. We would be running the same marathon on the same roads with these elite runners. Wow! There were no corrals or chip timing in place for this marathon; that would come in a few more years.

The weather wasn't bad, with temperatures of about 70 degrees with 70 percent humidity and overcast. There was light rain a few times during the marathon, but not as I ran through Central Park and to the finish. I will never forget the view running up the Verrazano-Narrows Bridge and through all five boroughs. I had never heard such crowd support at a race. My name was on my shirt and spectators were yelling out my name as I ran by. I thought the Marine Corps Marathon had great crowd support, but this was different.

The people were especially friendly as I was running through Harlem. They treated runners like celebrities. Women wanted us to touch the hands of their babies as we ran by. I took a few walk breaks even though I felt as if I were letting down the spectators when I walked.

When I arrived in Central Park I cried all the way to the finish. I was so happy. Running this marathon was the most incredible experience. It felt like a dream. The runners were handed their finisher medal and the women also received a red rose. I was happy with my finish time of 4:25:05. My low back did not bother me as I ran. In fact, my energy level was so high that I completely forgot about the pain.

I don't remember much about the awards ceremony that evening, but I do remember the place was loud and crowded. I decided to walk to TGI Fridays near the hotel for a cheeseburger and fries. I hadn't eaten much after the race, making that the best cheeseburger and fries I had ever eaten. I was wearing my finisher medal, and as I walked back to the hotel people came up to congratulate me and see the medal. I was happy to show it off and I didn't have a problem with anyone. The negative stories I had heard in the past regarding New York City just did not happen to me.

On Monday morning my legs were sore, but I could still get out of bed and walk. My low back really hurt at this point. If I had known then about the benefits of a warm Epsom salt bath I would have taken one. My train home left shortly after noon. I was thankful I could take my time and not rush, and I treated myself to a cab ride to the train station.

When I returned home I found the solution to my low back pain: a firm new mattress. Within just a couple of days I was a new person and that was the last time I have had issues with my low back.

10

Walt Disney Marathon #2
January 8, 1995 – Orlando, Florida

Destination races are great fun!
Look at races scheduled for anywhere
in the world you would like to visit,
and double your incentive.

I decided to sign up with Leukemia Team in Training for my second Walt Disney Marathon, along with eight other runners from the Annapolis Striders. On July 23, we started marathon training, following the training schedule for the Marine Corps Marathon even though we would be running Disney in January. I don't remember or have any notations in my running log that we had a special training plan for the marathon.

Participating with Leukemia Team in Training meant I was required to train with the group at least once a week. I still preferred to run on my own, so I wasn't happy with the thought of getting up early on Saturday morning for the 7:00 a.m. start.

But as I had discovered when training for New York, I really did enjoy running with this friendly group. This was an out and back training course along Route 450. There were trees on both sides of the road and once in a while we would see a deer or three. I soon looked forward to my Saturday morning runs with the group and getting up early was not as difficult as I had imagined. I would have a pasta dinner on Friday evening and retire by 9:00 p.m.

I was putting in high 40- and 50-mile weeks, with three 18-mile runs and a 20-mile long run. My low back was a little uncomfortable but otherwise I was pretty healthy. I still did very little stretching. I learned years later that stretches for the hamstrings and low back would take care of this problem. I was working full-time at a chiropractor's office and was on my feet all day. My runs were in the early morning before going to work and by evening I was too tired to stretch.

About 20 of us, including families, flew to Orlando on Friday morning the weekend of the race. My Annapolis boyfriend and his youngest daughter went with me. We checked into the hotel, the Dixie Landings, which was on the Disney property. After a little unpacking we were off to the Magic Kingdom for the rest of the day.

I spent most of Saturday at the Health and Fitness Expo at the Contemporary Resort and Convention Center. My running heroes, Mary Slaney, Joan Samuelson, and Alberto Salazar all signed my program, and I also met Greg Myers, and Bill Rogers for a second time. I still have my program, bib, and marathon shirt, and the Disney Marathon jacket I purchased.

The Marathon started again at Epcot at 6:05 a.m., following a beautiful fireworks display. We ran through Magic Kingdom/ Main Street at Mile 9, Mile 10, and Mile 17; Disney-MGM Studios at Mile 21; and entered Epcot at Mile 25. We also ran through Blizzard Beach, and ran past many of the Disney hotels. When we reached Epcot we started at one end of the countries and ran past all of the countries to the finish. I had a good run and my finish time was 4:17:37.

I finished the marathon number 45 out of 168 women in the age group 45-49. I was not a top three finisher in my age group, but I was happy where I finished. Placing in the top three in my age group was never a goal. I didn't think I could ever place in my age group in a marathon. That would come later, as I lost weight but gained more confidence and courage.

11

Boston Marathon Replay
April 18, 1995

If you think watching a marathon on TV would be boring, watch anyway. It could be the inspiration you need.

I watched the entire Boston Marathon coverage on ESPN the evening of the marathon. I had never watched this event on TV before. Some friends of mine from the Annapolis Striders Running Club were running, but of course I didn't see them on the replay. Boston was very exciting to watch even on TV though I never imagined myself running in that group of runners. April 18 would come to be a special day for me as well, for more reasons than one.

12

Time for a Change—
Once Again

Practicing self-care is not selfish.

Two weeks later, I found myself twice-divorced and having just ended a three-year relationship with my Annapolis boyfriend. I was now moving out of his house and looking for a roommate. I had answered several newspaper ads for roommates and met with several different guys. Each one was looking for a female roommate. I was more than a little suspicious and I asked each guy for their reason. They all said it was because women were cleaner and pay the rent on time. I decided to take a chance.

I moved into an old house in Eastport, just over the drawbridge from the City Dock in Annapolis. I had the upstairs. The house did not have air conditioning and very little heat in the winter. It was very rustic, and I loved it.

There was a swing on the front porch, where I loved to sit on Sunday mornings to have my coffee and read before going for my morning run. This was also a great place for people-watching. I had only lived on my own once before for only a short time, so this was a little scary, but also exciting.

> *If you are not happy where you are,
> take steps to change your situation
> until you arrive where you are meant to be.*

My roommate turned out to be a very nice guy and we were good friends for several years. He had a group of friends who came over to watch *Friends* on TV every week, and I would often join them. We had a good time together. Having a male friend was a real treat. We talked about everything. He felt more like a brother than just a roommate.

Eastport was a great area to live and run. I could run for miles and I felt very safe. I ran very early in the morning and there were plenty of street lights. I was close to downtown Annapolis and I could run through the Naval Academy. I was working a full-time job and running every morning, and I had plenty of time to read my books in the evening. Yet, I was still pretty lonely, especially on the weekends when my roommate would be off somewhere with his girlfriend. I wrote in my running log, "I will meet someone wonderful. I deserve someone wonderful, and he deserves me."

It was not easy to meet someone. There were several fun bars I could walk to from our place, but that got boring at times. Living the single life was proving to not be much fun for me, but I made the decision to not settle for anyone less than the person I felt I deserved.

I still missed my Annapolis boyfriend and we saw each other often. I knew he was *not* the one for me, but I was lonely and felt confused. After six months of separation, I moved back into his house. As I stood and watched the movers unload my possessions from the truck, I knew I was making a big mistake.

We stayed together another six months and then I moved out for good, back into the house in Eastport.

Two days later I saw him for the last time. When he came over to bring me my mail, he was high and I could tell he had been drinking a lot. That was it—my final wake-up call. I'd had enough. That little voice inside my head was screaming and I listened. I took the mail and yelled at him to never come back to my house or call me again.

It took a lot of courage to finally put myself first. As a child I was always told to put other people first, but the self-help books I was reading were telling me differently. It was time to put the old patterns behind me and try something different. I didn't like being alone, but all of that time to read and think had been helpful.

I was learning that it was not selfish to practice self-care. A friend told me to think about how a flight attendant, when addressing passengers, always says that if, in case of emergency, the oxygen mask from over the seat drops down, "…be sure and secure your own mask on your face first, before assisting someone next to you." Self-care is actually the best way to be able to help others, too.

That final-straw incident helped me understand once and for all how badly I had been treated all of my life. I had been taken advantage of, and physically and mentally abused by my mother and my first and second husbands. I had never insisted on the care and respect I should have expected. My Annapolis boyfriend did not physically abuse me but he was very selfish and self-centered. Still, I cannot regret this relationship because he was the reason I moved to Annapolis.

"Today, this ends," I pledged, "No one will ever mistreat me again." I had actually had a date with someone very special the night before, but at the time I did not realize just how special he was. I did not realize at the time that this was the man who would help change my life. It turned out that this was the man who would always be there to support me but would give me the space to figure things out when that's what I needed.

13

Roy—A New Beginning

There is a lot to be said for "partying with a purpose".

I had moved to Annapolis three years prior, to be with the boyfriend I had just left for the second time. I started to wonder if I should just give up on having the relationship I deserved and had been looking for. Maybe I needed to make some changes in myself first, and that was the very thing I did. I stopped blaming everyone else for my sadness and looked inside myself.

First, I needed to leave the past in the past. Next, I needed to forgive every person who had hurt me so I could move forward. This was not easy and did not happen overnight. I continued to read more self-help and spiritual books which were starting to wake me up. I knew I was holding on to a lot of anger and needed to let it all go.

I listened to many experts and read many books about the power of forgiveness. This was very new to me but was beginning to work. I did not meet with each person face-to-face; I was able to learn to forgive them through meditation. Today I do not hold a grudge against anyone who hurts me. I simply forgive and move on. It sure saves a lot of energy and sleepless nights, which allows me to be more present for the things that bring joy, like running.

> Reclaim your energy. Rather than waste time and energy on past hurts, anger, or sadness, learn to forgive and heal. You won't believe how much lighter you will feel!

I had been in therapy on and off for several years. One of the things I realized was that I had been trying to help the other person more than myself. I thought that if I could change the other person, then the relationship would be perfect.

I had started a new job at a chiropractor's office a couple of weeks before I moved out for good from my Annapolis boyfriends house. During a lunchtime staff meeting I mentioned that I have two passions, running and Jimmy Buffett music. After lunch, my co-worker Cindy told me that her husband's boss Roy was going through a divorce and he was a big fan of Jimmy Buffett. Could they give him my phone number? She thought Roy and I might get together and listen to some CDs and the relationship would not go any further.

Roy and I had our first date on May 12, 1995. He had tickets to an evening Buffett Booze Cruise that left from the Annapolis City Dock. I had heard about the cruise, but I did not have a ticket. Many of Roy's friends were also on the cruise and they were a fun group. I was actually more impressed with his friends than I was by him. The truth was that my Annapolis boyfriend was coming over the next day to bring my mail, and I was looking forward to seeing him (you already know how that turned out!). It's no wonder Roy and I didn't hit it off that night.

I knew I had messed up by not giving Roy a chance. When my roommate asked how things had gone with Roy on the cruise, I said he was okay and I'd really liked his friends. He suggested I give him another chance. I said he probably wouldn't be back because I didn't invite him in after the cruise and practically slammed the door in his face. Roy did not call me the next day so I figured it was over before it got started.

I was a member of the Baltimore Parrothead Club. A "parrothead" is a Jimmy Buffett fan, and through these clubs (there are hundreds all over the world) we celebrate Buffett's music and tropical spirit by giving back to our communities and having a lot of fun. Parrotheads "party with a purpose." I had told Roy and his friends about the club and our upcoming meeting at a restaurant called Fins, which was located in downtown Baltimore. Two weeks later, Roy called to ask if he could go to the meeting and if I would ride with him to show him the way.

That was a little over 23 years ago. Roy and I are still together and not only listening to Buffett CDs, but have been to over 40 concerts through the years. We were members of the Baltimore Parrothead Club for another year or so until two of my friends from the club and I formed the Chesapeake Parrothead Club. Since moving to Florida in 2005, Roy and I have been active members of the Space Coast Parrothead Club. It has become a wonderful lifestyle, participating with this group who parties with a pupose, making a difference to support causes from "Save the Manatees" to Alzheimers' fundraising. (Worldwide, Parroheads contributed in 2018 over 3 million dollars and over 200,000 volunteer hours.)

A special relationship, just like a marathon, means you have to be willing to take the first step, and then the next.

Roy and I were almost inseparable after the first night at Fins. Sure, we had some things we needed to work out. His three sons were young boys at the time and I wasn't sure I wanted to be a stepmother. My dream was to meet someone with a sailboat, not young children. The boys lived with their mother and spent every other weekend with Roy. I did not want to meet the boys until Roy and I were sure we wanted a committed relationship with each other. The weekends he had the boys, I really missed him and looked forward to Sunday evenings when he would come over after dropping them off.

After a few months Roy wanted me to meet his boys and I agreed. I was very pleasantly surprised at how nice all three were. The youngest had just turned eight and the oldest was twelve. All three had the most beautiful blond hair and bright blue eyes. The boys played baseball and basketball and Roy was their coach.

Roy really surprised me. I had never met anyone quite like him. He was nice, funny and responsible. He talked a lot. He seemed to be a very good father and I could see how much he loved his sons. When we'd watch a sad movie and I'd be crying my eyes out, he would actually get emotional too. This man was going to take a little getting used to.

When I met his mother for the first time she really sealed the deal for me. It was a Sunday afternoon and we took the boys to her house for dinner. Roy hadn't told me that his entire family would be there. I almost freaked out when I walked through the front door and saw so many people. His mom walked right up to me, put both hands on my cheeks and said, "I am so happy to meet you." Oh my God, I loved this woman. If she couldn't be my mother, I thought, I would certainly love for her to be my mother-in-law. To this day I tear up every time I think of our first meeting.

Christmas morning that same year, Roy gave me a Christmas card. Inside the card he drew a coupon which read, "This is good for one engagement ring." I said "Yes." I still have that card.

Roy and I were married September 29, 1996. Cindy was Maid of Honor and her husband Joe was Best Man. We are still great friends to this day. We were married at Fins in Baltimore, the same restaurant where we met with the Parrothead Club.

I loved our wedding day and cherish every memory I have today. It was a Sunday afternoon, with 50 of our family members and friends. The wedding ceremony included Roy's boys and my son in a special way that brought the family together. We'd discussed this with the boys ahead of time to make sure each one was okay with this and they were. Our Jimmy Buffett-themed wedding included cheeseburgers, fries and Margaritas at the reception, and each person was given a lei when they arrived.

I believe Roy is actually a divine gift, and I thank God every day—every hour—for this gift. No one in my life has ever treated me the way he does. He is loving, kind, thoughtful and considerate. I could see from the very beginning just how special he was, especially how nice he was to his mom and his three sons. He takes very good care of me; we take good care of each other.

The first few years we were together, I had a very difficult time getting used to someone being so kind. I still needed a lot of work on my issues. I told him when we first met that relationships are only good the first year. He was determined to prove to me wrong. I hate to be proved wrong, but in this case I am happy he was right. As the years go by I realize each year with Roy has been even better than the previous. Talk about a miracle.

When we reminisce about those early years, Roy tells me I had an edge. I wonder why he stayed with me; I was a mess. These days I am much softer and calmer. It took me a little time and Roy was very patient with me. I had told him everything I had been through and I guess he saw that I had potential. As I have said, he is a gift.

Every New Year's Day, we make plans for the new year. We write everything down and, at the end of the year, we look back at all of the good things that happened to us during the last 365 days. We look at the list we made at the beginning of the year and check off all of our accomplishments. We are very blessed and very grateful.

When I first met Roy, I told him I was serious about running and that he should never try and talk me out of running, including my early Saturday morning long runs. Roy has been my biggest cheerleader all these years. He is not a runner himself but he encourages me to run and race. Over the past few years he has organized a water stop at the Space Coast Marathon in November and the Melbourne Publix Marathon in February. I run the half marathon at both races and then join him at the water stop to help finish up.

On September 29, 1996, my last name changed to Kellner. I wear it proudly. In the book *26.2 Marathon Stories* by Kathrine Switzer and Roger Robinson, Chapter 4 describes the 1896 Olympics held in Greece. One of the 17 runners was the

Hungarian, Gyula Kellner. It's interesting that my running picked up when my name changed. Coincidence, or is there something in the name?

14

Marine Corps Marathon #5
October 22, 1995 – Washington, D.C.

Laughter is a wonderful thing!

This was my fifth and final time to run the Marine Corps Marathon. It was also Roy's first experience with me training for a marathon. According to my running log, my training was going very well. I was doing everything I normally did—I ran early in the morning before going to work, and on Saturday mornings I did my long training runs for the marathon. I was still running with my friends in the Annapolis Striders on Route 450. It was so nice to have water put out for us every two miles and I loved running the hills.

The Marine Corps Marathon started at 9:00 a.m. on a Sunday morning. I felt great during and after the marathon. According to my running log, the weather was perfect and there were great crowds. My watch finish time was 4:04:30 but my official finish time was 4:10:38 (this was still before chip timing). Roy was waiting for me at the finish.

The Marine Corps Marathon was 10 days before Halloween. That afternoon when we arrived back home after the marathon, Roy sat down to read the Sunday newspaper. He pulled out the TV section and on the front page was a picture of a werewolf in an ad for the movie *Frankenstein and the Werewolf.* Roy held up the picture for me to see, looked at me and said, "Jackie before the marathon."

I must have been a real monster and more stressed than I had realized the morning of the marathon. I cracked up laughing and I still laugh when I think about it today. Through the years my stress level has never gotten much better before a big race. He's just learned to deal with me. Thank goodness for his great sense of humor.

15

Walt Disney World Marathon #3
January 7, 1996 – Orlando, Florida

Finding perfection

My third Walt Disney Marathon was an experience I will never forget. One valuable lesson was to remember that even a breakdown can be turned into an adventure. I was joined by my friend Mary from the Annapolis Striders.

My training was going great. I ran almost every day. I was running the Annapolis Striders series races, along with 10-mile training runs on Route 450 Saturday mornings with my Striders friends all summer. Once again in the fall we began the Marine Corps Marathon training schedule. There are no notes in my running log about feeling sad or tired. That is a good thing.

After the Marine Corps Marathon on October 22, I started long runs again on November 4th, though now there were very few runners on Route 450 on Saturday mornings. Mary and I met up and it was nice to have a friend to train with, and that the water was still put out every two miles for anyone who was still training.

Mary and I flew out of Baltimore to Orlando on Friday, January 5, and everything went smoothly; we had a good flight, good weather, and an easy check in at the hotel. We stayed at the Port Orleans, a Disney hotel. We went to the Expo on Friday and Saturday and attended several seminars. On Saturday evening we attended the Carbo Dinner event at Disney's Contemporary Resort Convention Center.

I noticed in the program that more spectator areas were now listed. Yeah! Mile markers were listed where the spectators could watch. Walt Disney World truly is a magical place to be. I especially loved to run through Cinderella's castle.

Mary and I watched a little news and weather while dressing for the race, and heard that a major snowstorm was brewing in Baltimore. But we were having a great time in Florida where the weather was beautiful, and didn't think about the storm much at all.

The event started on Sunday morning at 6:30 a.m., again at Epcot. We started by running past all of the countries. Next, we were off to Magic Kingdom, Blizzard Beach, Disney-MGM Studios, and the finish at Epcot—once we ran past the countries for a second time.

I had a good run, though according to my notes I was a little tired at Mile 15. But I kept going and finished in 4:13:45. We now had a new technology called ChampionChip, where a chip was placed on the running shoe through the shoelaces. Now our finish times would be more accurate. I finished 31st out of 115 women in my 45-49 age group.

Mary and I arrived back at our room and were watching the Baltimore weather on TV while we showered and packed. We were due to fly back to Baltimore later that day, but things up north did not look so good. We decided to get to the airport and get out of Orlando as quickly as we could.

When we arrived at the airport the flight to Baltimore had been cancelled. We checked into a hotel near the airport, fully believing we would get out the next morning. Meanwhile, some of our Striders friends who had also flown down for the marathon had just rented a car to drive back to Annapolis. Unfortunately, Mary and I did not know this until a couple of weeks later. Not many people had cell phones at that time so we had no way of getting in touch. But after we arrived back home and spoke with our friends, we decided we'd had the more interesting adventure.

On Monday morning, we had breakfast and relaxed in the hotel room till around noon. Just the tops of my feet were sore. I never could figure that one out. After most marathons, for just a few hours, the tops of my feet are sore. Mary, on the other hand, had several blisters on her feet and was having a tough time walking.

We had a 4:00 p.m. flight to Charlotte, North Carolina, and things were looking up. We boarded the plane at the Orlando airport and were upgraded to first class, maybe because we were wearing our Disney Marathon race shirts and finisher medals. The flight attendant was so nice. When we told her about our situation she brought us each a bag of snacks. She was also very generous with the champagne. We were both working girls without much cash and were reaching the limit on our credit cards. These layovers were not in our plan.

When we arrived at the Charlotte airport, our connecting flight to Baltimore had been cancelled. We ended up sleeping on the floor at the airport along with other stranded travelers. I have seen this familiar scene on the news many times during the winter months, but I never thought it would be me. The airport staff provided everyone with blankets. I enjoy people watching but this was an entirely new adventure for me. Mary and I just tried to make the best of our situation.

On Tuesday we were still at the Charlotte airport, now in line to board a 1:55 p.m. flight to Baltimore. Just a couple of minutes before boarding time the flight was cancelled. I couldn't believe this. This wasn't fun anymore. Mary and I were having trouble reaching our husbands—the phone lines must have been down or all tied up.

Mary graciously offered to pay for a room at the Holiday Inn. Her credit card was approved so we were good for the night. We were in bed at 7:00 p.m. and slept for 12 hours. There was not much else to do but watch the news and sleep.

On Wednesday morning my credit card was approved for breakfast so we were in good shape, plus we still had snacks leftover from the plane ride from Orlando. We were once again booked on the 1:55 p.m. flight to Baltimore and this time the plane took off.

Roy was waiting for me at the gate and I was so happy to see him. I ran over and gave him a big hug and kiss. He felt wonderful. Mary's husband was waiting for her in their car just outside at the pick up zone with a dozen red roses.

Back in Annapolis the weather was much worse than I had imagined. I could not believe the amount of snow. Trucks were picking it up and dumping it into the Chesapeake Bay because there was no place else to put that much snow.

I was happy the trip was over. Still, Mary and I made great memories that will last a lifetime and I am grateful to have had this experience. I took a lot of pictures during that trip, especially at the airport. Once in a while I look at those pictures and I still smile—especially at seeing the lady that evening at the airport lying on the floor on top of her mink coat.

The day after I returned from Disney, Roy and I took a walk to downtown Annapolis to the jewelry store. We looked at diamond engagement rings, but I am not a diamond person. As we were walking out of the store I looked to the ring case on my left and saw a ring that caught my attention.

The band was gold with a stone in the middle of two smaller stones. The stone in the middle was tourmaline and the two stones on either side were amethyst. There just happened to be a holistic bookstore nearby, so we went and looked up the meaning of these two stones being together. We learned that these stones together are good for communication. Perfect! We went back to the jewelry store and Roy bought the engagement ring and gave it to me. To this day I still love this ring. The communication part really worked.

16

Key West, Florida
April 11, 1996

Nature's beauty can be a gift of running.

This was our first of many trips to Florida and the Keys, and it was all it took to convince me I wanted to someday move to Florida. Roy didn't want to move that far from his three boys, his mom, or his other family members in Maryland. For me, any Florida beach would have been fine.

For the time being I had to settle for frequent visits. My son, his wife, and our first grandson lived in Boca Raton, Florida, at the time. Over the next few years we flew to Boca two to three times a year and occasionally made the drive to Key West. Before Johnny and Gina moved to Texas they blessed me with two more grandchildren. Roy became Grandpa to the three. There is something so particularly sweet about seeing your child with their own children. I think it is a primal thing, perhaps because we see our legacy and gene pool continuation. I am just as proud of Johnny's parenting as I am of his Marine Corps and other accomplishments.

When my son was born, I decided that I would never spank him. I would look at that sweet face and no way could I hit him. Validation came soon thereafter as I was watching *Good*

Morning America on TV. A doctor, Dr. Haim G. Ginott, was talking about not spanking children. This advice was counter to what was typical thinking at the time. I purchased his book, *Between Parent and Child: new solutions to old problems*. This was a real eye-opener. I learned to explain to my son why whatever he did was wrong instead of hitting. After I explained three times, if he still asked why it was wrong, I gave up. "Just do it because I said so." But no beatings (like I had endured for years from my mother and grandmother.) Johnny has three children and he and Gina never spank. I know this because we talked about this several times and my son would always just tell me the truth; we have that kind of relationship.

After that one visit to Boca Raton when there was still only one grandchild, Roy and I left Johnny's family and headed south instead of north. I was very, very happy—we were on our way to Key West! Now, just because you are at the very southern-most spot on Florida's mainland does not mean you are that close to Key West. You've got at least another four hours to drive. We drove through the keys on the Overseas Highway (US-1). I love this drive. Once you pass the Last Chance Saloon you know you are in the Florida Keys. Roy decided to enjoy a shot of rum at each bridge. He had no idea just how many bridges there would be between the Last Chance and our motel in Key West! We made a pit stop at a Burger King and a guy in the car next to us was leaving the Keys headed back north…he offered us the last of his case of beer. Welcome to the Keys!

During this trip, I ran the 7-Mile Bridge Run, which started on Marathon Key. The weather was just beautiful with temperatures in the mid-70s, clear blue skies, and tropical breezes. I ran the seven miles over the bridge to where buses were waiting to bring the runners back to the start. The colors of blue and green in the expanse of water all around me were spectacular, and everything sparkled with sunshine. Runners had a time limit of 70 minutes to cross the bridge or be picked up by the bus. I finished in 1:00:02.

Roy was waiting for me at the finish but I couldn't find him. I finally heard someone yell, "Hey babe!" Roy had befriended the race director and was enjoying Jell-O shots. Our next adventure was the Duval Crawl, which was basically just going from bar to bar to stay cool. No details necessary… what happens in Key West stays in Key West.

On Wednesday morning, as we were driving to Miami for the plane ride back to Baltimore, Roy looked up at the sky and said, "There goes our plane!" I thought he was kidding but we were having such a good time we never checked our actual departure time. There's nothing better than getting stuck in Florida for another day! Unfortunately, we were able to take a later flight that day and the check-in agent accepted our story about the rental car breaking down. We figured she'd heard this little white lie before.

17

New York City Marathon #2
November 3, 1996

Endorphins and champagne go well together.

Mary and Margie, two of my friends from the Annapolis Striders, decided they wanted to run New York. We made a deal that we would all apply, but agreed that if one of us did not get in, none of us would go. On Friday, June 28, we each received our acceptance letters and started training the very next day on Route 450—we were serious about our training.

I was feeling better than I had in a couple of months and the notes in my log were much more positive. I can't find any mentions of feeling sad or tired. It looked like those days were over forever. Marrying Roy in September was a big part of that. We each had a new set of friends we really enjoyed spending time with, and life for me was getting much less stressful and worrisome. I have to also credit the fact that running is chemically beneficial to your mental health. Studies show that aerobic exercise can be as effective as anti-depressants, and for any runner, the endorphins released are just good for your mood.

I was also much more confident those days. I was now running 40 miles a week training for New York and I even had a couple of 50-mile weeks as we got into the longer Saturday training runs.

We decided to drive to New York rather than take the train, and Margie offered to do the driving. We left early Saturday morning. Our husbands looked sad that we were going without them. They had the opportunity to go but thought they would be too bored. We tried to look sad also, but as soon as we were far enough away we yelled, "Road trip!" and we were on our way to New York City.

We checked into the Park Lane Hotel, then were off to packet pickup and the Expo. We walked the entire day—first the Expo, then Central Park—any place Margie wanted to go. Margie had two small children at home and Mary and I teased her about not getting out much. After the pasta dinner at Tavern on the Green in Central Park, we took another walk through the park and then headed back to the hotel to turn in for the night.

My second New York City Marathon was just as exciting as my first. My official time was 4:24:17 but my watch time was 4:22:32 (this was still before chip timing). Margie and Mary were faster runners, which worked out well for me because by the time I arrived back at the hotel the shower was open.

We decided to skip the awards program and stayed in the hotel enjoying a bottle of champagne Margie had brought, sharing our experiences of running New York. Then I treated my friends to dinner at The Oak Room in the Plaza Hotel. A burger and fries cost $18.00 each but I did not care. I was with two great friends and we had just completed the New York City Marathon.

Monday morning was a real treat. We went to the NBC studios and stood outside with other marathon finishers during the

Today Show. I had watched this scene other years on TV, and now there we were!

We walked back to the hotel, packed, and headed back to Annapolis. This was a trip the three of us would never forget. Roy and I were still newlyweds and I was very happy to see him when I arrived home.

18

Walt Disney World Marathon #4
January 5, 1997 – Orlando, Florida

Find out what you've got in you,
what you're made of.

I was sticking to my goal to run the first five Disney marathons, so, come January, I flew like a migrating bird down to the south. This was also the twenty-fifth anniversary of Walt Disney World in Florida and the park was all decorated to celebrate, including Cinderella's Castle which looked like a huge birthday cake. Disney magic was everywhere.

I had signed up quite late for this one, on November 17. Roy said he preferred I go without him and enjoy the experience, without him being in the way. I am sure that if you are not a runner, all this Expo stuff and just watching people run for five hours is not very exciting.

My training went very well and I felt good most of the time. I was running my long runs on Route 450 on Saturday mornings, as usual. I was mostly running alone the last couple of months of my training since most runners had been training for the Marine Corps Marathon in November. The water was still put out for anyone still training for any upcoming races. The weather turned quite cold by December, down to 19 degrees one Saturday morning.

So many good things were happening in my life. I was still running all of the races in the Annapolis Striders Running Club series, and we even attended three Jimmy Buffett concerts that year. True Jimmy Buffett fans, Roy and I loved the beach lifestyle. One day we would have that all the time. For now, we were busy with family and friends—and our jobs.

I flew to Orlando on Saturday morning, very excited about the trip and escaping the cold Maryland winter. I checked into the Jamaica-themed Caribbean Beach Resort on the Disney property. Over the years this would turn out to be my favorite Disney hotel. I loved the colors in my room and there was a white sandy beach just outside. I could pretend I was really in Jamaica (in 2006 we would fly there for son number three's wedding). After check-in at the hotel, I was off to packet pickup and the Expo at Disney's Contemporary Resort Convention Center.

Race-day weather did not suit me, with temperatures of 70 degrees at the start and in the 80s by the time we finished. I was not used to that heat. It had been pretty cold at home in Annapolis during the last few weeks of my training. Unfortunately, I hadn't had the time to arrive earlier to acclimatize myself to the warmer weather.

I felt terrible the last six miles. I kept thinking to myself that this would be my last marathon. I wasn't happy with my finish time of 4:38:39, which was number 59 out of 181 women aged 45-49. I am sure other people who came down from the north had issues with the heat also.

I still have the official picture of me crossing the finish line and receiving a slap of the hand with Mickey, framed on the bookcase in my running room. As I was running and getting closer to the finish line I could see Mickey Mouse congratulating the finishers with a slap of the hands. I was so tired I just didn't feel I could hold out my hand. At the last second I managed to touch hands with Mickey, but I was looking down. I just wanted to get over the finish line. Other finishers in the photo look as drained as I do.

As I noted in my running log, this marathon helped to show me what I am made of. I wrote in my running log, "I am not quitting the marathon. I'll just get better and enjoy the accomplishment." When I wrote this I had no idea just what the future had in store for me.

19

Walt Disney World Marathon #5
January 11, 1998 – Orlando, Florida

*Feeling sometimes like a warrior,
sometimes like a wimp—
this is normal.*

I had decided. The Fifth Anniversary Walt Disney World Marathon would be my last. Not just my last Disney marathon but my last marathon—period. I planned to continue running half marathons and shorter races.

My training was not going well. It was a very cold winter and Roy was traveling a lot with his job. He was away mainly during the week and would be back home Friday evening or Saturday morning. I missed him.

One high point during this time came on October 26 when my oldest grandson, Dakota, ran his first race. He was about three years old at the time. It was a 50-yard race and he came in First Place (took after his grandma!). I was so proud. Today Dakota is 23 years old and has graduated college with his master's. He recently completed Marine Corps Officer's Training at Quantico in Virginia, finishing first in his class in athletics, and second in academics as well as in leadership. I can't wait to see what his future holds.

After the Marine Corps Marathon I was alone on Saturdays for my long run once again, and I missed running with my friends. The water was being put out every two miles. Some runners were probably out before 7:00 a.m., as I would sometimes see a few runners as I approached the turn-around and headed back to the start. It was on one of these long Saturday runs in December when I tripped and fell soon after I started out. It was dark when I started and I was probably not paying attention. When I got up and got myself together I almost turned around to go back to my car and call it a day. But I kept going instead. After I arrived home and took off my running tights, my left knee did not look so good. I cleaned it up and there had been no pain when I ran so I got on with my day.

Over Christmas, Roy and I both had the flu. We'd both had flu shots but we still ended up very ill. We lay around the house all day Christmas Day. My temperature was 102 degrees. I hated to miss spending the day with family, but both of us felt terrible and did not want to pass on that flu to other family members. I felt much better by January 9 and I flew to Orlando (two days before the Disney race). Roy hadn't come with me and I didn't know if any other Annapolis Striders were there. But my goal was to complete the first five Disney marathons, so there I was. After checking into the Caribbean Beach Resort once again, I went to packet pickup and the Expo, which was now held at Disney's Wide World of Sports complex.

Over the two days, I attended several seminars, including one about women's road racing hosted by Joan Samuelson, and another hosted by Frank Shorter. One that I *didn't* attend was "The Boston Marathon: A Winner's Look Behind the Scenes," hosted by Alberto Salazar and Amby Burfoot. If I only knew then what I know today…I can't believe I missed that one! But I definitely did not think I could ever qualify for the Boston Marathon so why would I attend the seminar?

I met Bill Rogers for a third time at the Expo on Saturday and he signed one of the books he co-wrote with Priscilla Welch. I had met Priscilla Welch at a race in Virginia shortly after the book was published and she autographed it for me, but it took a few more years for me to meet Bill. He wrote, "Let's always run. Follow Priscilla's advice." I met Bill once more at a race in 2009 after we moved to Florida and he signed the book again. This time he wrote, "You're still running." Yes, I took your advice, Bill. Thank you.

Sunday morning, my hotel phone rang and it was Mickey. I loved hearing Mickey's voice for my 3:00 a.m. wake-up call. I got dressed and caught the bus that took the runners to the start at Epcot. The marathon started at 6:00 a.m. and we were seeded based on our estimated finishing time.

The weather was perfect at the start, with temperatures in the 40s and no wind. The sun arrived shortly after the race began. Sunrise is one of the things I loved every time I ran this marathon. I ran slowly just for the pure enjoyment of this marathon, feeling a little sad that this would be my last Disney Marathon (I learned after this to never say "never again," because I just don't know what the future may hold for me).

I wanted to enjoy every mile, but each mile seemed to go by much too fast. I felt good the entire 26.2 miles and finished in 4:50:58, which was number 112 out of 256 women aged 45-49. I had now completed my goal of running the first five Walt Disney World Marathons. I would miss not coming back the next year, but it was now time to set different goals.

When I arrived at the Baltimore airport the following afternoon, Roy was there to pick me up and I was so happy to see him. The weather was certainly not what I had left in Florida, but I still felt good and I started running again on Friday. I was still not taking the advice to take one day off from running for each mile of a race.

During the rest of 1998, I mainly ran the races in the Annapolis Strider Championship series, in which I placed first in my age group. I also ran the Bay Bridge 10K and the Annapolis 10-mile race. I ran very few long Saturday morning runs on Route 450 with the Striders. I was enjoying getting up a little later on Saturday morning and running from my house. Most of my Saturday training runs were less than five miles, unless I was training for a longer race. It was nice to take a little break from my normal routine, but by summer it was hot and humid and, basically, I had turned into a wimp.

I would turn 50 in December and I was not looking forward to that. There were very few runners over the age of 50 in the Striders, so I felt my running days were just about over. I was almost finished going through menopause, which was good news for me and everyone who lived with me, but I was still trying to figure out how to lose the extra weight that had come along with it.

Roy went all out to celebrate my fiftieth birthday, which made me feel much better. The first time I saw a Ford Mustang was when I was in high school and I knew one day I would have one. I still have the 1998 Mustang convertible Roy gave me for this birthday. He also took me to New York City to see the Christmas Show at Radio City Music Hall and we stayed the night at the Plaza Hotel. Turning 50 was not so bad after all.

Roy and I also bought our first house in 1998. Setting up the house was keeping me busy along with working full time. To my surprise, I found that I enjoy doing yard work. I just like being outside. I planted flowers in the spring and then fall flowers at the end of the summer. While there were three guys living in our home, I was the one who liked cutting the grass.

20

My Florida Dream Comes True
Our Move to Florida – 2005

Running enhances life.
Running is not life. Keep a balance.

My dream had come true and we were on our way to Florida. Roy had wanted to wait until his youngest son graduated from high school, and I wanted him to be absolutely sure about the move.

We had spent the past two years checking out different cities in Florida. My first choice was Key West but that was too far from family. My son and his family had lived in Boca Raton for several years, but by then they had moved to Texas.

Roy sat down with a map of Florida and drew a line through the middle from the Gulf to the Atlantic. Places below the line would be too hot most of the year. Places above the line could be colder than we wanted during winter months. Roy is very practical. I just wanted to move close to the beach.

We also made a wish list: close to a major airport in case of a family emergency; close to the beach but not on the water; and driving distance to Key West. And, of course, close to Walt Disney World. We also wanted a town that was not too big, or too small. Being from Atlanta and Roy being from Baltimore, we agreed we wanted to absolutely avoid highly congested areas.

We purchased a townhome in Palm Bay, on the Atlantic side of Florida. On Saturday, August 27, 2005, both cars were packed and we were on our way, stopping for two nights in Savannah, Georgia.

Neither Roy nor I were retiring at this point. I had worked in the medical field for many years and was able to find a job pretty quickly once I had the house unpacked. Roy had switched from the corporate world to real estate a few years earlier and found employment also. I joined the Space Coast Runners, and Roy and I joined the Space Coast Parrothead Club.

The townhouse was in a good location for my early morning runs. A ball field with restrooms and water was only a couple of miles away. I ran my first race on November 20—a 5K that I finished in 27:56, placing first in my age group of women 55-59. There were actually many men and women here over the age of 50 still running and racing, making this a great start to the next phase of my running.

A lot of good things happened after the move in 2005. I was running races in the Space Coast Runners Club series and placing in my age group in almost every race I ran. My motivation was high and I was loving the weather. I was getting used to the heat and humidity and loving both. It was so nice to not have to bundle up in the winter months. Florida is a state for sunshine lovers, and I was *at home*. I was running in shorts and a jog bra; I would have never run without a shirt in Maryland. I stayed nice and tan all year long.

My Florida lifestyle included running, but Roy and I work at keeping everything in balance. After a few years I was running 14-16 races each year and we were also busy with the Parrothead Club. We've made many new friends through this club and are more involved with this one than the previous two. As I mentioned earlier, the purpose of a Parrothead Club is to "party with a purpose" and give back to the community. Our club collects food for the Sharing Center, baby diapers for the Women's Center, and school supplies for the Grandparents Raising Grandchildren program. We also donate toys at Christmas, clean up the beach, restore dunes by planting sea oats—I don't know of any organization with such a variety of ways to contribute.

We love Jimmy Buffett's music because most songs are fun and very upbeat. We started to have more parties at our house and join friends for parties at their homes. Some of our favorite parties are the backyard concerts where local trop rock (tropical rock) performers are invited to sing and we all chip in to pay for the entertainment. We also bring a dish to share, chairs, and of course our drink of preference. For me, running is enjoyable, but it also helps me stay healthy so I can enjoy many other opportunities in life. Running is my thing, but it's not my *everything*.

21

Walt Disney World Marathon #6
January 13, 2008 – Orlando, Florida

It's hard to quit Mickey at any age.

This was the 15-year anniversary of the Disney Marathon. I had said *no more marathons* but here I was once again. I had tried to sign up for the half marathon but it was full, so I took that as a sign. I was 59 years old and in the 55-59 age group.

My training went well, although I was still not using any specific training schedule. I was trying to get used to the heat and humidity here in Florida. Since I was between jobs, I did my long runs alone during the week. I found a park a few miles from our townhome that had restrooms and a water fountain, and I would carry a small paper cup to fill up with water to stay hydrated.

I was still using *The Complete Runner's Day-By-Day Log and Calendar*, and 2008 was the Thirtieth Anniversary Edition by Marty Jerome. For 2008 my goals were: run 26.2 miles per week – check; run all races in the 2007-2008 Space Coast Runners Runner of the Year (ROY) series – check; place in my age group of women 55-59 for the series – check (placed 3rd); Disney Marathon – check; Space Coast Half Marathon – check.

Roy and I drove to Disney on Saturday morning. I was excited that we now lived this close to Disney, only about an hour's drive away. We stopped for packet pickup at Disney's Wide World of Sports Complex. After exploring the Expo (Roy actually went with me), we checked into my favorite lodging on the Disney property, the Caribbean Beach Resort, one of their Jamaica Hotel rooms. As usual, I had pasta for dinner, then retired to our room to relax and massage my legs and do a little stretching. Roy went to the hotel pool bar to watch sports on TV.

It was difficult to get to sleep and stay asleep and I was happy to finally hear Mickey's voice on my 3:00 a.m. wake-up call. The bus picked up the runners at the hotel to take us to the start, and most of the runners were pretty quiet and looked as sleepy as I felt.

In the past, the marathon and half marathon events had started at the same time, but now the half was run on Saturday and the full on Sunday morning. The marathon start was now broken down into corrals, according to your estimated finish time. I was in Corral F. I was honest with my estimated finish time, but I was sure many other runners were not because of how many of them I was passing.

No matter how many times I visit Disney I still get very excited—the kid in me comes out. Running through the park with the spectators cheering is the best. My finish time was slow but I was happy. I said many years ago that if I could not run a marathon in under five hours I would give up the marathons. My finish time was 5:15:44 and I finished 43rd out of 186 women in my age group. Not bad, but now it really was time to finally give up the marathon, or so I thought.

22

Walt Disney World Marathon #7
January 11, 2009 – Orlando, Florida

Do not worry about being a runner and getting older.
Age is just a number if you are healthy.

I definitely remember why I signed up for this one. Roy was kind enough to point out that I had a streak going: I had run a marathon in my 30s, 40s and 50s and by January 11, I would be 60 years old. (Thanks, hon, I love you too.)

Roy made a big deal about me turning 60. At breakfast on my birthday he gave me a card, and inside was a coupon for a night at the Breakers Hotel in Palm Beach. If you have ever seen this hotel you would know this is a big deal. We stopped in there for a drink a few years earlier when we were visiting my son and his family. We sat at the bar to have a drink, where they have this extraordinary aquarium full of small fish. The aquarium is actually the bar. I had never seen anything like it and we talked about how it would be nice to come back sometime and spend the night.

I had a 5K race that Saturday morning, and right after that we drove the two hours to Palm Beach, where we were promptly upgraded to an oceanview room for no extra charge. It was so beautiful I wanted to stay in the room until check-out time the next day, but we ventured out for dinner in the hotel restaurant. The hotel was decorated for Christmas and looked so beautiful. I had another wonderful birthday.

I started training for the Disney Marathon on September 27th. I was finally following a 16-week training program I had read in *Runner's World*, called "Marathon Training for Busy People, Running by Time." I thought I could follow this one.

I was still training on my own. I prefer Saturday morning long runs rather than Sunday, while the Space Coast Runners schedule their long runs for Sunday mornings. Sunday morning is my special morning with Roy, and it is good for me to take a break from running at least one day a week.

I got in most of my long runs, though I took off a couple of Saturday mornings from my schedule to run the Space Coast series races. One of these races was the half marathon Thanksgiving weekend. I like this race but I had a difficult time placing in my age group that year, finishing 9th out of 46 women in the 55-59 age group with a time of 2:18:32.

My sweet husband always makes our travel arrangements. I asked him several times over the months if he had made reservations at a hotel on the Disney property. Each time he said he would get to it and that it would not be a problem to get a room. He procrastinated until it was just about time to go. He said there would still be rooms available—but he was wrong. Only the most elite Disney properties still had a few rooms available, so he booked a room at the Hilton outside the park. Now I needed to figure out how to get from the Hilton to the start. I could have Roy drive me to the start but it was now too late to figure out the route to the drop-off.

I was assured when we checked in that there would be a bus to take the runners to the start because there were other guests in the hotel who were also running. The morning of the marathon I went to the lobby and saw other runners looking as confused as me. We needed to get to the start and there was no bus to take us, but there were several cabs out front. There was no time to waste so five of us decided to share a cab. The driver assured us that he knew how to get us to the front gate of Epcot.

The driver did not realize that many roads would be blocked off to drivers, leaving only one path to the entrance to Epcot. It was now too late to turn around and get into the line of cars that were dropping off runners, and we were all getting very nervous. We finally found a spot at Epcot that looked like it was near where we should be. We probably walked 20 minutes to the holding area. I had just enough time to check my bag at bag check, stop at the ladies room, and arrive at the start just in time. (My husband has never made the same mistake again.) Roy met me at the finish and seemed very happy that I actually made it to the start of the race.

This was another great marathon. *I can still do this,* I thought. I finished a little faster than the previous year—5:13:25, which was sixteenth out of 92 women in my age group 60-64. I was not just getting older, I was getting better.

But now, I told myself, this really was my last marathon. Training for a marathon was getting more difficult, plus I had told myself a few years earlier that I would give up the marathon if I could not finish under five hours. This was now the second time I had finished a marathon over five hours.

I decided to focus on races no longer than a half marathon, and that is exactly what I did for the next four years. I liked the shorter races. I figured I could continue to compete in the Space Coast Running Club series, and maybe run races in other Florida cities or other states. Maybe we would combine a vacation with a race. I didn't know what the future held for me.

23

Health

Make it first place in your life.

Nourishing and exercising your body is the foundation for all accomplishments, great and small.

I have been very fortunate to have good health over the years. I have actually become healthier as I've gotten older, especially after moving to Florida. In fact, I recently got a concerned call from my insurance company because it was August and they'd only received one claim from me. I explained that I do not get sick and that my chiropractor, for which the insurance company does not reimburse, takes very good care of my health.

I have had very few minor injuries due to running, like a heel spur, plantar fasciitis, and sciatica. One thing I learned from the heel spur was the importance of getting a second opinion. I was living in Annapolis at the time. After the first podiatrist examined my foot, he told me to give up running and that the heel spur would never go away. That was not good news, so I sought out another doctor.

As she examined my foot, I talked the entire time about my running and how much running means to me. She patted my foot and said, "Let's get you back on the road." I don't remember the treatment, but the heel spur was not an issue after a few weeks and has never returned.

Since developing a good stretching routine before and after I run I have not had the same issues again. Before I run, my routine includes sit-ups, push-ups, hamstring and other leg stretches. After I run, I also do something called the Tibetan Rites, which are a series of five yoga stretches completed 21 times each. I learned about them on the Dr. Oz show, and you can google it to learn more.

On the days I don't run, I do those same exercises plus I add hand weights. While I love full body massages I don't have them very often. Mostly I massage my own legs and take Epsom salt baths.

I do take a tumble every couple of years or so. My feet will just go out from under me or I'll trip on something. I have never had a serious injury or broken bone from a fall, just a bruised ego and skinned knees and hands.

Weight was a recurring issue for much of my life. I thought I ate pretty healthy when we lived in Maryland, but I was going through menopause at the time and my weight crept up to 148 pounds. A gynecologist discovered a fibroid on the outside of my uterus, which was about the size of my fist. He suggested a complete hysterectomy.

Fortunately, I also spoke to one of my co-workers and she referred me to a holistic nurse practitioner who specialized in female issues. I liked her immediately. She examined me and spoke with me for an hour. I had never had a medical person spend so much time with me. She asked about my relationship with my husband and reviewed my supplements. She suggested we keep an eye on the fibroid and that I shouldn't worry because the weight would come off.

The weight would come off? This was a professional telling me this. I always thought that women were doomed to gain weight with menopause. *Did I hear her correctly?* Not only did the fibroid shrink, but the weight started to come off. And, I still have all of my female parts.

I had first started receiving chiropractic care in Virginia, when I first got serious about running. In Maryland, I worked for chiropractors for several years and learned more about the body and how to take care of mine. After moving to Florida, I tried several different chiropractors but hadn't found one that I wanted to stay with until I met Dr. Michele Munnich in the spring of 2010.

A good chiropractor who also focuses also on nutrition can be profoundly helpful.

Dr. Munnich also does nutritional testing, which revealed my gluten sensitivity. She suggested I switch to gluten-free products. Eating gluten free does not guarantee weight loss but it is working for me. I must have been eating more wheat than I realized.

My basic Medicare policy does not pay for the care I receive from Dr. Munnich. Since I pay her out-of-pocket, I decided to follow her instructions. I also gave up my one diet soda each day and switched from eating ice cream most nights after dinner to eating it once or twice a year. After making these changes my weight dropped to the lowest I can remember—117 pounds—and I've stayed there. I may gain back a couple of pounds after holidays and pizza, but they come right off within a few days.

The best part is that I don't starve myself and I don't count calories. I believe that what I put inside of my body is most important. My husband tells our friends that I eat more than he does and he is right. I eat three meals a day, mostly vegetables and very little meat, and I don't snack between meals except for a yogurt after I run. I have also lost my sweet tooth. There was a time I enjoyed baking cookies and cakes, but these days I usually only bake at Thanksgiving.

The only food I really crave is the lunchtime salad I eat almost every day. It includes avocado, black beans, and brown rice, along with romaine lettuce, broccoli, and tomato. I do also enjoy two pieces of dark chocolate after lunch.

Losing and keeping off the weight is making a difference in my running and, especially, my confidence. Another bonus of my chiropractic care is that, at 69 years of age, I have never had knee or joint issues. I may have good genes, but I believe I am in good shape due to stretching and chiropractic adjustments. My chiropractor checks me out once a month and keeps my body in balance. She also reviews the wear on my running shoes for any imbalances. I purchase new shoes as often as needed—usually at least four pairs per year.

Because reading is very important to me and I want to continue to have good eyesight, I also have my eyes examined once a year.

I have not had any skin issues but I rarely use sunscreen. So with all the time I spend outside running, working in my yard, and going to the beach, I knew it would also be a good idea to start seeing a dermatologist every year. At my last appointment the dermatologist told me I have really good skin, so I've decided to save the co-pay and let my husband examine me instead (he prefers to do this more than once a year—wink!).

Sleep is very important. I'm normally in bed by 9:00 p.m. and up at 6:00 each morning, and some days I'll rest in the afternoon.

I don't take prescription drugs. I had a cyst removed from my right thumb in 2004 and the nail also had to be removed. When the doctor gave me the prescription for the pain pills I asked if I could have a glass of wine with the pills. He said no. When Roy came home from work I was sitting in the den watching TV with my right hand propped up and a glass of wine in the left hand. I was feeling just fine and never needed the pain pills.

I never was a smoker. My husband smoked until after his first son was born then gave up cigarettes for good. No one in our immediate family smokes. Thank you, family. God gave me this body. It is my responsibility to take care of it.

24

Race Day Routines

Good pre-organization ensures calmer nerves on race day.

If you have run a race or two and felt like a fish out of water, believe me when I say it gets much better. You will develop your own practices and routines that work for you and make you feel confident and calm. My race day routine starts the night before. I eat a pasta dinner before every race or long Saturday run. I've also learned over the years to set everything out the night before. I gather up all of my small items and pack them into my RooSport pouch, which clips onto the waistband of my shorts.

I don't wear a water belt because there is normally plenty of water and Gatorade offered along a course, so I am always well hydrated. Into my pouch goes lip gloss (I don't leave home without this!), a protein bar, which I can take in small bites while I run and I know it sits well in my stomach, and four or five CLIF BLOKS™ Energy Chews, which I just let melt in my mouth as I run. These are designed for people training and racing, and are offered in many flavors including orange, black cherry, citrus, and even margarita!

Breakfast is one slice of gluten-free bread with peanut butter and strawberry jam, one boiled egg, and half a banana. I drink water with a little PowerAde mixed in as I travel to the start, along with two cups of coffee.

I've read for years that after a race it is good to take one day off for each mile run, but I have never needed to take that much time off. Listen to your body and don't rush it.

I am not sure when I started the following practice to get me thru a marathon, probably after the move to Florida. I am very good at staying very focused while I run a marathon. At the start of the race I do not think about running 26.2 miles. My goal is to get to mile 20 without a walk break. At mile 13 I think – only a half marathon to go. I have run many half marathons so I know I can do this. With 10 miles to go I remember running 10 mile races so I know I can run 10 miles. With 6 miles to go I know I can run a 10K. With 3 miles to go I know I can finish a 5K. With the last mile I think – just 4 times around a track. Before I know, I am across the finish line.

I do wonder at times if I don't push hard enough in the races. I am never so sore that I can't walk or climb stairs after a marathon. But my plan is to run and participate in races for as many years as possible. I think that if I push much harder I could get injured and my running days would be over. I do what my gut tells me to do.

If I get up in the morning and don't feel as good as I would like, I know that once I start stretching all of that will change. It is rare I don't feel like going out for a run. I love the Nike slogan—"Just Do It." I read once that if you don't feel like running, go outside and get started. After a few minutes, if you really don't feel like a run that day, then turn around and go back home. At least you tried. A wise person once suggested

I make the decision to exercise one time, then just keep doing it. Don't try to make the decision every day. That made a lot of sense to me.

I started a morning meditation practice after moving to Florida, at first using a weight loss meditation I saw Deepak Chopra demonstrate on The Doctor Oz Show. Now I incorporate stretching and running as part of my meditation. As much as I love to listen to music, I do enjoy the quiet time of meditation, plus this allows me to pay attention to my surroundings and listen to the sounds of nature as I run. I focus on my form and on any upcoming race. If I'm struggling with any issues, I work these out on my runs as well. It's amazing how often solutions come to me as I run.

I ran listening to music for years but gave it up before moving to Florida. I don't run with music, I run with positive thoughts and this gets me into a peaceful meditative state. Each morning, as I start my run, I thank God for another beautiful Florida morning. I also say, "Thank You that I am having a good and safe run." As I run I continue saying to myself, "I am blessed, thank You."

As part of training, practice thinking positive thoughts and encouraging affirmations. This will help on race day when you start to feel tired.

25

Our Move to Melbourne

*Good is the enemy of best.
Don't settle, find your rainbow!*

We lived in Palm Bay for six years, but I was not happy with townhouse living. The housing market had been very tight in this area when we were looking, and the development met our needs and moving schedule, but I found that I really missed taking care of a yard. We didn't have the boys living with us anymore, so there wasn't as much to do at home to keep busy. I changed jobs several times during those years in Palm Bay, and in-between jobs I slid into the habit of sitting all afternoon, watching TV. I realized that our townhome and the area were not as condusive to an active lifestyle as I would like.

Most of our activities and new friends were several miles further north from where we lived, so when we decided to move, we looked in the Melbourne, Florida area. We spent two years learning about all the communities and homes for sale, and were happy to see the housing prices were starting to drop. This would be our final move for many years, so we decided to take our time, and it was well worth it. We moved in 2011 and both love the house and community we decided on. Even though we were over 55, we did not want a 55-and-over community. Instead, we now enjoy a family community with residents of all ages.

We are not on the beach side but just a 10-minute drive away. We have a short jaunt over the Pineda Causeway to A1A, and to the left of A1A is Cocoa Beach. To the right is Indialantic. Every once in a while, on a Sunday, we drive to Indialantic for a slice of pizza at Bizzarro, and then an hour-long walk on the beach. Melbourne Beach and Satellite Beach are also nearby.

We are not far from the Kennedy Space Center at Cape Canaveral. When rockets are launched from the Space Center we can walk out our front door and see them go up. First you see the brightness, then the billowing trail. Day or night, it is an awesome sight. Then we feel the ground rumble, even though we are about 30 miles from the launch pad.

We are now in an HOA community. A lawn care service cuts and edges the grass, but we were given the option of maintaining our own plants and shrubs and I choose to do that. For me this means more exercise and sunshine, much better than afternoon TV! Plus I am learning more about tropical plants and how to take care of them. Our home looks very tropical inside and out. (Jimmy Buffett would love it!)

There is a lake behind our house with turtles, fish, ducks, sandhill cranes, otters, and all sorts of interesting birds—but no alligators. At least, that's my story and I'm sticking to it! And, of course, we have lizards (we prefer to call them geckos) that live on the front porch and the back porch, but seldom come in the house. I have seen an occasional deer at the lake and in other areas in the community. I know from other runners that Florida also has panthers and bears, but I don't think any are in our area.

We are three houses away from the community pool and playground. I love the sound of children playing. We are only a couple of blocks from Home Depot where I can buy plants and anything else I need for the yards. I can run safely for many miles starting just steps from our front door. Wickham Park and the Running Zone store are less than two miles away. I am very happy here.

As of August 12, 2012, my days of employment were over, although I don't consider myself retired—I feel busier now than when I worked full time. The big difference is that I am doing more of the things I want to do, like volunteering with local charities. I was Membership Officer for the Spacecoast Parrothead Club for two years, then Community Service Director for four years. Roy served two two-year terms as the club President. I am a morning person so we are still up each morning at 6:00 a.m. It is best to get out for a run early, before it gets too hot. Roy plays golf at least once a week. We find that most "retired" people here lead surprisingly active lives.

I love living near the beach and in an area where it is warm most of the year. At least six months out of the year we don't need air conditioning. We open the doors and windows and let in the fresh air. In the winter months, if we run the heat two weeks, that is a lot. A tropical breeze flows through the house most days. Every morning when I wake up I feel like I am on vacation.

Some mornings we get up early and go to the beach for sunrise. I don't remember paying much attention to clouds before moving to Florida, but the clouds are so beautiful here. A Florida sky can be bright pink, golden, purple, orange, and all shades in between. During the rainy season in the late afternoon, I see some of the most spectacular rainbows I have ever seen. I spend much more time outside these days than ever before.

26

Walt Disney World Marathon #8
January 13, 2013 – Orlando, Florida

How you train makes all the difference on race day.

Here I was again, this time because it was the 20th anniversary of the running of the Disney Marathon. When I saw the ad in *Runner's World,* and the picture of the awesome finisher medal, I knew this one was just too good to pass up.

By this point my weight was down quite a bit and I was feeling great. I used another *Runner's World* training program, "Your Best Marathon Plan" by Janet Hamilton and *Runner's World* experts. The long runs were scheduled for Sunday so I had to do a bit of juggling.

I was now doing my long runs over the Melbourne Causeway on Saturday mornings in order to get in some hill training since the area where I live is pretty flat. I parked my car at Front Street Park (this park has restrooms, which is handy!) and started my training runs at 8:00 a.m. by running four miles, first through downtown Melbourne (out and back) and then over the Causeway.

I can get in a lot of miles on the other side of the Causeway before turning around and going back over the Causeway and to my car, plus there are two water fountains on the other side of the bridge. Often other people are out for early morning runs and walks, too. The water view from the bridge is always beautiful, especially if there are dolphins to watch.

Training days passed quickly and it was time to head to Disney World. Roy and I were both grateful that we were so nearby now, instead of having to fly down from Maryland. He and I drove to Disney on Saturday morning and went straight to the Expo to pick up my race packet and check out some of the vendors. Then we checked in to the Caribbean Beach Resort, Jamaica Hotel (still one of my favorites). After a pasta dinner, I relaxed in the room and Roy went to the pool bar to watch a football game.

The morning of the marathon, my reliable and punctual friend, Mickey Mouse, woke me up with a phone call at 2:30 a.m. and I got ready to catch the bus to Epcot for the start. Knowing the course so well has its advantages—I knew exactly which restroom to visit to get in and out quickly after entering the Magic Kingdom.

That was the only break I took. I ran the rest of the course without a walk break. I had learned from running past marathons that I don't like walk breaks. It is difficult for me to start back running, and I feel lazy. Once I take a walk break I just want to take more walk breaks and I get tired rather than push through. It messes with my mind to take a walk break, though I'm sure for some people it serves a purpose and is energizing rather than tiring.

The temperature at the beginning of the race was in the 60s, and it was 80 with 100% humidity by the time I reached the finish. I now trained year round in this heat and humidity so I was not as affected as in earlier years. Just one more benefit of living in Florida!

I had never eaten a banana during a half or full marathon, and couldn't stomach the thought, but my energy level was dropping just as I finished running through All Sports—I saw a table piled with bananas and took one. I ate it slowly, and I was relieved that it sat well in my stomach. Plus, it tasted great and seemed to give me a little mental boost, too.

I must have been at least considering the Boston Marathon at this point because on the back of the running training schedule I had written down the 2013 qualifying time for women 65-69, which was 4:40. I was very happy with my finish time of 4:59:19, which was 18th out of 179 women in the 60-64 age group. My weight was down and my finish times were coming back down also.

I still have the article from *Florida Today* that talks about the number of runners from Brevard County who ran this Disney Marathon—194 of us. I finished 24th out of 102 women, most of whom were younger than me, and only four of us were over 60. Of those four, I came in First Place. I felt very proud, and after a short break I was running again by Saturday.

27

Boston Marathon Bombing
April 15, 2013

Stay strong.

I watched the beginning of the 2013 Boston Marathon on TV, then went out for a training run. I came back home and watched until the TV coverage was over, though the marathon was still underway. I had some shopping to do so it wasn't until I had returned home and turned on the TV that I saw the news: at 2:50 p.m., two bombs exploded in a crowded area near the finish line.

Like so many other people trying to absorb this horrific news, I was in shock. I needed to talk to someone, but Roy was working so I called a friend. We were both watching the news and couldn't believe what we were seeing.

I kept thinking that this just does not happen before, during, or after a race. This should be a happy time for so many people, runners and spectators alike. I know what it's like to cross the finish line at the end of running 26.2 miles. No matter how tired I feel, I am exuberant. A marathon event is normally very celebratory for all.

I continued to follow the news over the next couple of days as I took time to let the tragedy sink in. I think I was in such denial that this could have happened that I needed to keep watching. Gradually, it became less surreal, and more upsetting. Three innocent people were dead, hundreds more injured.

Looking back, I believe this was when a seed was planted in my heart and soul that I would like to try to qualify for Boston. While Boston was never on my bucket list, something inside of me had changed. That little voice was speaking loud and clear. My qualifying time for Boston had to be a 4:40 finish and I had finished my last marathon in 4:59:19. That was a lot of time to take off. *I don't know about this*, I thought, *I'm not getting any younger...*

When my July 2013 issue of *Runner's World* arrived it was a special issue about the bombing. I read the issue from cover to cover twice, taking in the stories and photos. I cried both times. I can still feel the pain of that day. But many things had happened since the day of the bombings that helped begin the healing process, and one that really touched me was the impact of just two words: "Boston strong". An expression of Boston's unity after the bombings, the slogan showed up on T-shirts and other products, and was emblazoned on the wall at Boston's Fenway Park. The Boston Bruins displayed the slogan on their helmets at their hockey game two days after the bombings, and at the first baseball game in Fenway Park after the bombings, the stadium announcer told the crowd: "We are one. We are strong. We are Boston. We are Boston strong."

In that same *Runner's World* issue, there was a marathon training plan by Amby Burfoot called "A Foolproof Marathon Training Plan." It was a 20-week training guide, which looked a little different from other plans I had reviewed over the years. The long run was planned for Saturdays, which I preferred.

I made copies of the running schedule so I could take notes and still preserve the magazine. I still have my copy of the plan folded inside that year's running log.

I would be in the 65-69 age group for Boston 2016, and my qualifying time would be 4:40. I assumed that if I qualified I would be confirmed to run (which is not always the case), but this was all new to me so I needed to study all the rules.

I had already signed up for the 2014 Disney Marathon, so my opportunity was right in front of me. I wasn't sure I could run a qualifying time (4:40) but I needed to stay positive. I knew that if I didn't believe I could qualify, there was no need to even try. As so many have said before, *if you believe it, you can achieve it.* I had to drop the "if" and use positive self-talk, especially during my training runs. It works!

28

Walt Disney World Marathon #9
January 12, 2014 – Orlando, Florida

Get your mindset dialed in to
YES, I can do this!

This was my ninth time running this marathon and I knew the routine very well. I felt ready. I had started Amby Burfoot's 20-week training the week of August 26 and it had gone very well.

Roy and I drove to Disney on Saturday morning and checked into the Caribbean Resort once again, opting for the convenience of staying at a Disney property. I had a relaxing evening in the room, but I still had a hard time falling asleep. I often have stressful dreams about an upcoming race, like I can't get to the start line for some reason, or the starting gun is about to go off and I am not dressed in my running clothes or can't get my running shoes on. I've had dreams where I am hopelessly lost on the course, or I'm on my hands and knees and trying to pull myself to the finish line. Luckily, I get through all my worst-case scenarios in my sleep, not during a race, thank goodness!

On marathon morning I was up at 2:30 a.m. for the 5:30 a.m. start. I still loved that Mickey would call to wake me. It was a perfect morning—cooler than I had expected, but I was dressed just right. It had rained hard during the night but was clear by morning. I never overheated during the race and I did not take any walk breaks.

As I ran through All Sports, I was getting hungry and my energy was getting low. I remembered there had been a table of bananas the year before and, thank God, there it was again, piled high. I took one, ate it very slowly, and it worked for me once again.

It was a good race. Roy met me at bag check and I ran over to him and gave him a big hug and kiss. My finish time was 4:44:48—better than any previous time, and just 4 minutes and 48 seconds over my qualifying time for Boston. I was so excited I was sure I would burst.

I had to wait until I got home that afternoon to see my official finish time posted online, where I also saw that I placed second for women 65-69. I yelled for Roy to come look because I was sure it had to be a mistake. I checked the results an hour later and again the next morning, just in case.

I never imagined I would place in my age group in a marathon, especially a major race like that one. There were 46 women in my age group and I missed first place by only seconds. I still look at my finisher medal and the letter I received from Disney, both displayed in my running room. I am so proud of what I have accomplished. Each accomplishment you have, big or small, can be used to dial in your mindset, to get stronger and firmer in your belief, "YES, I can do this."

Roy and I talked at length about the possibility of me qualifying for Boston and he encouraged me to go for it. Thank goodness he is so supportive. I don't know if I could have pursued it and perservered, otherwise, since I did not have a coach and I was doing my Saturday long runs alone instead of with a group.

I decided I was going to run Boston so I needed to take more than 4:44 minutes off my time to qualify. Some people suggested that I enter as a runner for a charity, which would have meant I didn't need to meet the qualifying time as long as I met the fundraising requirements. But I preferred to meet the challenge and get in on my own running ability. I was not afraid; my confidence was at an all-time high. I *believed* I could *achieve* this goal.

On February 2, I ran the Publix and Melbourne half marathon and placed second in my age group. There were only seven women in my age group, but second is second. I felt great and my running was going very well. I continued with my 10-mile training runs on Saturdays unless I had a race. I did well through the summer, even in the heat and humidity. I only stopped for water and didn't take walk breaks.

Mid-July, I started marathon training for the Space Coast Marathon scheduled for November, using Amby Burfoot's training plan for the second time. I normally run the half marathon but I chose the full distance just for this year.

This would be a good marathon for me to qualify for Boston. I knew the course has only rolling hills, it is close to home, and my husband and friends would be working one of the water stops. This was my opportunity to "go for it" and I had the right mindset, which always makes all the difference.

29

Space Coast Marathon
November 30, 2014 —Cocoa, Florida

*Focus on your plan and
do not have a back-up plan.*

It was almost 6:30 a.m. and I was lined up to start the Space Coast Marathon. This was the marathon I had chosen to qualify for Boston. It was now or never. I had no backup plan. I just don't think that way.

The start of the race was in downtown Cocoa Village. The street lights were on as well as the storefront lights, but this was no time for window shopping—I was very focused. I had run the Space Coast Half Marathon every year since 2006 and I knew the course well. The marathon starts north, makes the turn and runs to the south end, makes another turn, then heads back to the finish (the half marathon just covered the south end of the course).

For the past several years, Roy had organized the water stop at the turnaround at the south, and there would be more than 20 of our friends from the Parrothead Club there with him. I had also worked it out with Roy to have a banana waiting for me but I warned him there would be no time for chatting. "Just hand me the banana and I will see you later."

The Space Coast Marathon is always held on the Sunday after Thanksgiving, which makes it not an easy one to run. I do most of the Thanksgiving cooking, which I look forward to each year, and we invite a few friends to help with the feast. After that, though, I try not to eat too much until after race day—of course I still have my usual pasta dinner the night before the race.

This is a very well-organized race, managed by the owners and employees of Running Zone, our local running store. There were many familiar faces I knew from the Space Coast Runners group, running both the full and half. The race began with a video of the Challenger taking off from the nearby Kennedy Space Center.

I am very careful when selecting the pacing group I start with at the beginning of a race. I had planned for months to start with the 4:40 pacer. I found the 4:40 pacer and was waiting patiently for the race to start. Seconds before the start of the race a little voice inside told me to move up to the 4:30 pacer. I really needed to run a little faster than 4:40 just to be on the safe side because I knew that Boston only allowed 30,000 runners.

At 6:30 a.m. we were off. I was feeling great but there was a little problem. The 4:30 pacer was running the Jeff Galloway walk/run plan. This would be fine except the runners in the group were taking up the entire right side of this narrow road and weren't moving over to the right when they stopped to walk. I couldn't stay in front of the group because I didn't want to burn too much energy running faster this early in the race, yet I also didn't want to stay behind the group.

When the group took their walk breaks it really affected my pace. I needed to slow down in order to avoid running into the person in front of me. I was wasting much needed energy and time. A girl I knew from the running club was running next to me. She was not happy with the situation either but we didn't know what to do.

I had been meditating for several years and had learned to be patient, and just breathe. I couldn't afford to waste precious energy that early in the race. I tried to stay to the left of the group as much as possible and went around them each time they stopped. I just needed to be careful once we turned around on the north end, because some of the slower runners in the marathon were still coming towards me.

I was feeling good and having a great race. I was almost at Mile 20 and had not taken a walk break. I got to the south end and Roy was waiting with my banana. He wanted to peel it for me but I grabbed it and kept going. I didn't have time to waste, and I'd warned him earlier there would be no talking.

Seeing my Parrothead friends at the water stop and listening to them cheer for me really perked me up. The motivating cheers and my banana will now get me to the finish. The view of the Indian River to the right is very beautiful but I kept my focus on the road in front of me.

I stayed with the 4:30 pace group until the turnaround at the south end of the course. That is when I start to slow a little. We only had about six miles to the finish. I ate my banana slowly and perked up. A couple of miles before the finish I started to get tired. I kept telling myself that I was in the lead, *I am first, I am first*. I took a few very short walk breaks before the finish. I knew I was still in good shape time-wise.

A Boston Marathon Journey

The finish of this race is always very exciting for me. We finish in Riverfront Park next to the Indian River, which has a beautiful view of the Merritt Island Bridge. There were so many spectators at the finish and they were cheering very loudly for the runners. This was not the time for any more walk breaks; there were too many people watching!

I crossed the finish and my official finish time was 4:36:10. I placed 1st out of 10 female runners in my age group of 65-69. I should have been thrilled about my finish time but I was tired and it hadn't yet sunk into my brain. I accepted the beach towel which was given to the runners as they finished, along with my finisher medal. Then I needed food. The finish always has plenty of food for the runners like pancakes, eggs, pizza, and fruit. After I ate and picked up my checked bag, I waited for the awards to be given. It sure felt great being called up to the stage and given the award for First Place in my age group. I had now placed twice this year in my age group in a marathon. That was never on my bucket list. And, I qualified for Boston. My head was spinning, and I hadn't even drunk the free beer!

I called Roy to have him pick me up. The finish and the water stop are six miles apart and I was not walking! He needed to stay with the other volunteers and work the water stop so he had our friends Laura and Chuck drive out to get me. When I got in the car I was so excited I was talking non-stop. When I told them I'd qualified for Boston they both looked confused.

Somehow Roy had the impression that I hadn't qualified, and he'd asked Laura and Chuck not to say anything to me about it because I would be upset. After they realized I had qualified they were very excited for me and we all had a laugh.

I thought I'd told Roy when I called him that I had qualified but apparently he hadn't heard me. It can be very loud at the water stops with all of the cheering. It actually turned out better that way because I got to tell him in person and I got a great big hug—even though I didn't smell so good. He was so happy for me. Placing first in my age group made all of the hard work even sweeter.

Over the years I have read articles in *Runner's World* and books about runners who wanted to qualify for Boston. Many go through a lot just trying to qualify. They go to specialists, and do all sorts of special training, such as speed work. I did very little special training and I didn't have a coach.

I still believe one of the main factors that got me there was losing the extra 30-plus pounds I'd been carrying. Also, that I am very disciplined and focused. I have a very positive attitude and believe in the power of affirmations, of "I am." Adding to all of this the support and encouragement from Roy did not hurt.

Later that day I turned on Oprah's *Super Soul Sunday* and I heard a wonderful quote that I wrote down in my running log: "If your dreams aren't big enough to scare you – they aren't big enough." I didn't catch the name at the time, but this phrase was also part of the Harvard 2011 commencement address by Ellen Johnson Sirleaf, former Liberian president and the first elected female head of state in Africa. What a perfect thing for me to hear that day.

The 2015 Boston Marathon was already filled. This was November 2014 and I would have to wait until September 2015 to sign up for Boston 2016. I had no idea how stressful the wait would be.

In the meantime, I finished the 2014/2015 race season for the Space Coast Running Club. It was my best race season ever. I had placed at Disney and placed and qualified for Boston at the Space Coast Marathon. At the spring banquet for the running club I received three awards: Female Senior Grand Master, Ran all Races in the 2014/2015 series, and Placed First Female Age Graded.

At the April 12, 2014 Space Walk of Fame 8K I set a course record for Female Senior Grand Master. My time was 46:54. I was very proud of myself. It was just a small local race, but this was another first for me.

> "Whether you think you can, or you think you can't—you're right."
> —Henry Ford

30

Sign-Up Day for the Boston Marathon
September 21, 2015

Every epic journey starts with one first step.

Once the Boston Marathon opens for registration, runners with qualifying times sign up on different days according to their finish time. Monday was the first day to sign up if you were 20 minutes or more under your qualifying time. On Wednesday, you could sign up if there were any spots open and if your finish time was 15 minutes under your qualifying time. On Friday, if there were any spots open and you were 10 minutes under your qualifying time, you could sign up.

I kept my fingers and toes crossed all weekend because, if there were any open spots remaining on Monday, I could sign up. By Monday morning, I was about to lose it. I was very excited and very nervous. If there were any openings left, and if I was 5 minutes under my qualifying time, I could sign up online. I found that there were still spots available but I had no way of knowing just how many. I was very careful as I filled out the application. I did not want to make any mistakes, and I asked Roy to double-check everything for me. I sat for a minute thinking about the possibility of being accepted, and then I hit the "submit" button.

Now all I could do was wait. I had no guarantee that I was in. Registration would close at 5:00 p.m. that Wednesday, and the instructions stated it could take up to 60 days to get a *yes* or *no* answer. I was very happy my wine cooler holds a case of wine; I figured I might need it.

I couldn't get the confirmation off my mind. I checked my e-mail every chance I got, and Roy snuck on and checked occasionally, also. I exercised and ran every day, which helped relax me—somewhat.

The running season for the Space Coast Running Club had started, and I was running 10 or 12 miles on Saturday mornings for my long run. I had signed up months earlier for the Space Coast Half Marathon which is held the Sunday after Thanksgiving. Since I had my coveted qualifying time under my belt, I chose the Half Marathon rather than the full one that year.

Yes, I was waiting on my registration confirmation, but I was not *sitting around* waiting. I trained, practiced positive self-talk, and kept my diet aligned with my belief that I would be running in the Boston Marathon. Though nervous in a way, I just had a good feeling about it. And, there was the gift of today, this moment of life to enjoy. I didn't need to hold my breath as if life was on hold. Besides, it was time for some romantic R&R with my husband.

31

Cedar Key, Florida
Our 19th Wedding Anniversary

Taking time to relax should not be optional.

Now that we lived in Florida we had been visiting a different city in Florida each year for our wedding anniversary. In 2015, for our nineteenth anniversary, we went to Cedar Key on the Gulf of Mexico side of Florida. I knew nothing about Cedar Key, but Roy had read about it and wanted to go there.

We arrived to find it was a very small island and did not seem to have much to do (we learned later that we were there a couple of weeks before fishing season, which was the best time to visit). We checked into the Cedar Cove Resort, where our room had a view of the Gulf.

Unfortunately, the weather was not cooperating. It was overcast and drizzling—not the right weather for water sports, or the boat trip Roy had booked to another island. There weren't many stations or cable on the TV to watch. I had a couple of magazines but no books, and there was no bookstore on the island. *God help me.*

On the morning of our anniversary I made coffee and we sat on the patio to watch the sunrise. These had been the best 19 years I'd had in my entire life. In the distance was a lightning storm dancing across the sky—amazing, and so beautiful. We could see the Gulf and the lightning storm in the distance, but there was no rain. The tide was out and we watched a crab swimming in the shallow water. It was pure bliss.

The rain that did come was only slight, off and on, so I ran each of the two mornings we were there. Roy went for walks. We went for more walks together in the afternoon just to explore the island and look for any shops that may be open.

For our anniversary dinner, we chose The Island Hotel on the main street. It was a bed and breakfast with 10 guest rooms and a restaurant. It was a good choice. We had a delicious meal and we even ordered cheesecake. We don't eat dessert very often so this was a treat, and in honor of our anniversary, the cake was on the house.

After my initial disappointment about the weather and things being so quiet, I made the decision to just relax and make the most of our time in Cedar Key. I like to stay busy so slowing down is not always easy for me, but all in all we had a nice couple of days. Roy is so much fun to be with and it turned out he is the only entertainment I really need. For dialing back the fast pace that life can crank up to sometimes, Cedar Key is a good choice. I noticed that on the second morning of running, I felt more relaxed overall than I had on the first day. This fit with our intention for R&R, to enjoy one another and celebrate not only our anniversary, but our amazing life together.

Wondering about my Boston confirmation was not always top-of-mind, but neither of us forgot about it for any length of time. When I signed up for Boston, I had put the charge on our credit card. Roy didn't tell me this, but every day after I'd signed up he checked to see if the payment had processed. He knew that would be a good sign I was "in" because Boston probably didn't give refunds. Every day he saw the payment just sitting there "pending" and he didn't know what that meant.

On Monday before we'd left for Cedar Key, he checked the credit card account one more time. The payment was not showing in pending and did not show in paid. He was confused but didn't say anything to me. He was concerned the payment had expired but decided not to call the card company to check. He would just wait and see what happened.

Wednesday morning arrived and it was time to start our trip back home. I checked messages using my phone. Oh my God, my confirmation from the Boston Marathon had come in!

I had to read it a couple of times and then have Roy read it. I had been accepted into 17 previous marathons but this one was different. I was shocked, very happy, crying, and I didn't know what to do next. I wanted to get out of the car and jump up and down. Roy was all smiles. Talk about the perfect way to top off our anniversary celebration!

Once we arrived home, I had to read the confirmation again and I printed a copy from my desktop computer. A full packet of information arrived in the mail a couple of weeks later.

Roy did not waste any time booking the hotel and airline for our trip to the 2016 Boston Marathon. He was almost as excited as I was.

I think my chiropractor, Dr. Munnich, was the first person I texted from the car before we even left Cedar Key. "Keep me healthy. I am going to Boston." Next, I texted my son, and then my friend Cindy. After that I just went down my contact list.

But there was someone I knew I wanted to tell in person. Shortly after we got back home from our trip, I drove the mile or so to the Running Zone, our local running store, and asked for Denise. She and Don were the race directors of the Space Coast Marathon and owners of the Running Zone. "Is there something I can help you with?" asked the clerk, but I told her I had something to show Denise.

When Denise came out from her office, I handed her the confirmation letter without saying anything. She was so excited she gave me a big hug. I told her I was especially happy that I had qualified at the Space Coast Marathon, a race she had directed. As the founder of an organization supporting running in our community, I knew she would be happy for me in a different way than my family and friends were. It made me realize how running clubs, training partners and coaches, and participating in road races can build a powerful comraderie.

On November 29, 2015, I ran the Space Coast Half Marathon. I had run the half every year since moving to Florida, except the previous year when I ran the full and qualified for Boston. In 2015 I finally placed in my age group. I placed second for women 65-69, with a finish time of 2:17. There were 67 women in my age group that year. I was on a roll.

32

**Training for Boston
November 30, 2015**

And, just like that—"training" became "training for the Boston Marathon".

The very next day my marathon training began. It was time to get serious because April would be there in a flash. Once again, I was using the Amby Burfoot 20-week program. It had worked for me twice in 2014, once for the Disney Marathon and again for the Space Coast Marathon, and I was very comfortable with it. Luckily, the first week was very easy, just three miles each day for four days. This gave me a bit of a rest after the half marathon I'd just run.

33

Publix Florida Half Marathon
February 7, 2016 – Melbourne, Florida

Obtacles that are mountains to some are mere molehills to the determined.

Now the pressure was really on and I got serious with my training. Though I'd decided to forego the races in the second half of the Space Coast Running Club series to focus on Boston, I had run the Publix Florida Half Marathon every year since its inaugural event February 8, 2009, and it fit well into my training plan.

It was not the best morning for this race and the temperature and wind were considerable factors. The temperature was much cooler than normal. A lot of runners didn't show up, but I'd paid my money so I was there. Standing around waiting for the start was the hardest part, though I also had a hard time running on the Melbourne Causeway. I felt as if I would be blown off my feet several times. I was happy when this one was over.

My finish time was 2:22:26 and I came in First Place out of the 10 women in my age group of 65-69. As usual, placing in my age group in a race was worth all the work and hassle.

I did not run the next day but got right back on my training schedule Tuesday morning. According to my running log, my training seemed to be very uneventful. The weather was never an issue, since our rainy season is not until April. I actually enjoy running in light rain as long as the temperature isn't too cool.

During a few training runs in the past, I had tripped and fallen. Twice I've had to jump over a snake that I did not see until the last second. Thankfully I have never had a serious injury from a fall—just injury to my pride. As Boston got closer, the pressure was on during each run to stay on my feet. Luckily, since I was retired now, I no longer needed to run early in the morning before daylight (so the snakes were easier to spot!) and I could take a short nap in the afternoon if needed.

My Saturday morning long runs through downtown Melbourne and over the Melbourne Causeway were going well. As my training progressed, I continued adding miles through the communities on the other side of the Causeway. I'd finish running the last two miles back over the Causeway and return to my car.

My Boston Marathon opportunity started to feel so real, so close that I could almost reach out and touch it. Rain? Heat? Potholes? Snakes? Nothing was going to be a deterrant, now. If a mountain would have sprung up in front of me, I would have just included it in my training for that day.

Before leaving for Boston, my running friends, my Parrothead friends, and my family and neighbors were all wishing me good luck. As a treat for myself, I went to get a full body massage. At my last chiropractor visit before I left, my weight was at 116 pounds, my body was in balance, and I felt great. Dr. Munnich asked if she could say a prayer for me and I agreed.

We sat down facing each other, and she took my hands and said the sweetest prayer. Tears were rolling down my face. She had helped me greatly over the past several years and I appreciated her so much.

I was excited for Boston, and about as ready as I was ever going to be. I had done a lot to prepare for this—even an average runner like me can do what it takes if they are determined. Now, I felt strong in mind, body, and spirit.

34

The Boston Marathon
Boston, MA – April 18, 2016

Yes, I can.

Roy and I flew from Orlando to Boston on the Saturday morning before the Monday marathon. I was up early and ready to go, having laid out my clothes and bags the night before.

Everything went smoothly at the airport. I checked a bag but carried on one small bag with my running clothes and shoes for Monday so they always stayed with me—advice I had received years ago. Airports had never lost my luggage and this was not the time to have my luck change.

We had a good flight. Roy slept while I read marathon tips in *Runner's World* magazine for probably the hundredth time, and anything else I'd thought to bring. I was too wired to sleep.

I didn't know how many people on this flight were going to Boston to run the marathon, but just as we landed the pilot said, "Welcome to Boston and for those of you who are running the marathon, good luck." Well, I just about lost it. I can tear up and get emotional at times, and this was one of those occasions. This was just the start of a trip that could have not been more perfect.

We were staying at the Marriott Courtyard in the Theater District, which was within walking distance to all of the places we wanted to see. The weather was beautiful, with temperatures in the low 60s and sun. We only needed a light jacket to keep warm.

After lunch we headed to Boylston Street for packet pickup, which was at the John Hancock Sports & Fitness Expo. On the way, we stopped at the finish line of the Marathon and I just stood and stared. I felt as if I was in a dream. I had a hard time believing I was there and this was really happening. The area looked so much smaller than it does on TV.

I took some time to think about the bombing that occurred on that same spot three years before. I looked around at all of the people gathered who were smiling and laughing, and I thought about the people who were killed or injured that day. In my mind's eye I could see the faces of some of the people who were there as I remembered the survivors' stories I had read. I said a prayer for everyone who was at the finish line that day.

We went on to the Expo and I picked up my race packet and t-shirt. It was really crowded. I realized I was doing too much walking and standing ahead of the Marathon but I wanted to get to as many vendors as possible. This was a once-in-a-lifetime experience for me and I wanted to take it all in. What I really wanted to get my hands on was "the jacket." For years I have seen people proudly wearing their Boston Marathon jacket and now it was my turn.

I did manage to find Amby Burfoot, who was there doing a meet and greet. I showed him my copy of his training plan and told him his plan had gotten me through two successful marathons and I had used the same training plan for Boston. He wrote on my plan, "Jackie: Run strong. Amby Burfoot." I still have this tucked into my 2016 running log.

After four-and-a-half hours at the Expo it was time to go back to the hotel and figure out where to go for dinner. I do love to eat and my three meals a day are very important to me. We found a restaurant around the corner from the hotel and it was packed with a line out front. I did not write down the name of the restaurant in my running log but I did state that I had a wonderful salad. We lucked out on a table in the bar area and had a delicious meal, and we were back at the hotel and in bed by 7:30 p.m. after a very full and special day.

For breakfast on Sunday, Roy found The Paramount on Charles Street. They had four- and five-star reviews and had been around since 1937 so we decided to give it a try. Roy happens to be excellent at picking good restaurants and this was no exception.

Now, I am not a very large person at 5'2" and 117 pounds, but I can eat. I ordered gluten-free waffles with fresh strawberries. I also ordered scrambled eggs which came with potatoes. Roy ordered his own breakfast—I was not about to share mine. It was the best breakfast I'd had in a very long time, and it was easy to understand why the restaurant was so popular.

Runners can enjoy big wonderful meals, guilt-free!

It was time to walk off that big breakfast. We were near the Harbor so we started there. We also walked through Boston Commons, and stopped by the bar where *Cheers* was filmed. I purchased a wine glass for a souvenir. After we finally arrived back at our room we shared a veggie wrap and lay down for a while. Roy dozed but I was too excited to sleep.

I knew I should be getting more rest but, again, this was a once-in-a-lifetime event for me. I had never been to Boston so everything was new to me. I was not planning to re-qualify for Boston or run a specific time. I just wanted to finish the marathon and I knew I could do that, so I decided to just enjoy the trip and the race.

After all of the years I have been running I still eat pasta before a race or Friday night before my long runs on Saturday morning. We decided not to go to the official pre-marathon pasta dinner; Roy suggested we head to "The North End," an Italian section of Boston, instead.

Our food was out of this world. The restaurant had gluten-free pasta, which I prefer. As usual, I left very little for the garbage. We had planned to take a cab back to the hotel, but we were so stuffed from this delicious dinner that we walked back instead.

I was grateful there wouldn't be a 4:00 a.m. wake-up call like there are for some marathons, but we were still back in our room and in bed at 6:30 p.m. We watched some TV to relax, then turned in for the night.

I slept very well that night, which was unusual for me the night before an event, but I was happy to wake up on race day feeling great. I was both excited and nervous and was trying to keep myself calm. This was also Roy's 67th birthday and he had plans to go to Fenway Park where the Red Sox were playing the Toronto Blue Jays. It would be his first time at Fenway Park and he was looking forward to the game. He's always loved baseball, having played in high school and coached his boys when they were young. He had a great time, and there were lots of people to talk to—Roy makes friends very easily.

Packing clothes for a marathon is never easy. I had brought a long-sleeved shirt, a tank top, and a regular running t-shirt. When I checked the weather it was calling for 56 degrees and sun. The long-sleeved top could be too warm, and the tank top too cool the closer I got to the finish line. I decided on the t-shirt, with running shorts and compression socks. There would not be a bag check at the start and I knew I'd need a little something on my arms to stay warm as I waited for the start of the marathon.

I didn't have a long-sleeved running shirt I was willing to toss, but Roy had brought an old long-sleeved shirt I could wear until just before the race started and leave there. Roy is much taller than I am so the shirt looked more like a dress on me. Discarded clothing was being collected for the homeless.

After breakfast, Roy and I walked to The Commons where I would catch my shuttle for the start. We arrived at the park in plenty of time and we sat on a bench for a while until it was time for me to go to the bus. I was getting a little nervous and Roy was anxious to get to Fenway Park for the game.

I found the shuttle I was assigned to and got in line. Roy gave me a big hug and kiss and left me with, "See you at the finish. Run fast. I love you!" I started chatting with another lady who was also in line for the bus and we decided to sit together. We talked the entire way; you can get to know a lot about a person during a 26.2-mile ride. She was from Houston, Texas. My son and his family lived just outside of Dallas at that time so we had something in common besides being in Boston to run the marathon.

While the conversation made time fly in a way, the bus trip seemed very long. Block after block, through traffic lights, turns, shopping areas, residential areas…I kept thinking, *I've paid good money to get off this bus and run this long way back.* It is no wonder non-running friends think I am nuts! Eventually we arrived in the small town of Hopkinton and disembarked.

We hung out in Athletes' Village which was at Hopkinton High School and Middle School. Runners who had arrived earlier left behind large pieces of cardboard. My new buddy and I sat down on one to rest for a few minutes, and we took a couple of potty breaks before heading over to the start line. I knew I would not be stopping again for a potty break once I was on the course. It's allowed, but not in my mind.

I was in the fourth (yellow) wave, Corral 3 & 4. The walk to the start line was .7 miles. It was a slow walk. I had assumed the security would be tight, especially around the finish, but I was not prepared for the number of uniformed snipers standing with their rifles on top of the small buildings. This did not concern or frighten me; I was fascinated by everything I saw.

I took off Roy's shirt on the way to the start. There were already people bagging the discarded clothing and loading the bags into a truck. It was a beautiful morning and I was very comfortable. I had made a good decision with my running outfit. The temperature did start to cool a little around Mile 5 near Framingham, but I was still comfortable.

At the start, I stood and looked around at the other runners. Then I looked to my left and saw a small church. I remember saying a prayer that I would have a good race but most of all a safe race.

11:15 a.m. was a late start time for me. I was normally at the finish of previous marathons or getting ready for lunch around this time of day. I remember thinking, *God I hope I can do this*. Then I very quickly told myself, *Yes I can*. And then off we went!

The pack was a little tight at the start. Within seconds we ran down a very steep hill. I felt I needed to slow down and take shorter steps so I would not stumble and fall. This was not the time to take a tumble. I was not prepared for this. I'd been warned that the first 10 miles were mainly downhill but this was a little more "down" than I had expected. I had heard much more about Heartbreak Hill, which was near the end of the course.

I remember running through towns like Ashland, Framingham, Natick, Wellesley, Newton, and Brookline. We ran on fairly narrow two-lane roads, closed off to traffic. I was surprised by how much support there was from the crowds. Men, women and children stood cheering us on. Each town was like a big party with families and neighbors lining both sides the streets, some even having cookouts on their front yards. I thought the course would be fairly quiet until we ran through Wellesley and down Boylston Street to the finish. Thankfully, I was wrong. Even in the sections between the towns there were people cheering.

In the past when I ran a marathon, my goal was to get to Mile 20 before taking a walk break if I needed one. This day was different. I took my first walk break before the half. I had a good six hours to finish so I was still in good shape. I was not worried about not finishing so I took a walk break any time I felt I really needed one.

I tried to run up most of the hills. Normally I was a good hill runner and looked forward to an occasional incline. I don't even remember running up Heartbreak Hill, though I do remember a couple of long hills. I found out later that it was between Miles 20 and 21, just past a bridge we ran on that took us over a highway, and that it's called Heartbreak Hill because it comes so late in the marathon. I was just focused on getting to the finish at that point. I do remember seeing the John A. Kelley statue, located about a mile before the base of Heartbreak Hill. John Kelley completed the Boston Marathon 61 times and finished first place twice. He is a beloved icon of the Boston Marathon.

I had always heard about the female students at Wellesley College and how loud they cheer. I could hear the cheering well before we approached the school and there were banners of encouragement all along the road barrier. I passed the area much faster than I would have liked. It would have been fun to hang out for a while or turn around and run past one more time. Thank you, ladies, for the support. It was even better than I had expected.

I was getting pretty tired, but I was enjoying the Boston Marathon so much that I wasn't sure I wanted the 26.2 miles to end. I kept telling myself that this was a one-time deal for me and to enjoy the experience and keep running until I cross the finish. I was looking forward to seeing my husband and telling him all about my experiences.

I was also getting hungry; it was now well past my normal lunch hour. I had the thought that a banana might perk me up. Just then I saw a table on the side of the road with people handing out peeled half bananas. I didn't care if it was clean or not—it was a banana and I grabbed one, and this did help to perk up my energy.

Around Mile 23 or 24 I could tell we were getting close to the finish. Instead of small towns there were now office buildings, apartments, and condos. I could see the city of Boston in the distance and it was getting closer. The crowds were also getting much thicker, and so was the security. The security personnel seemed to be standing shoulder to shoulder at this point. I still felt very safe.

I was now at the last stretch before taking the left turn onto Boylston Street and to the finish. I could see the left turn not too far ahead. I decided to take one last walk break so I could run down Boylston Street to the finish. There was no way I would take a walk break on Boylston Street. I wanted to finish strong.

I took the last left turn and now I could see the finish. The spectators were much louder than before. It was now late in the marathon but there were still many people here cheering. I made it to the finish, too tired to even cry with emotion. I ran through the finish and finally stopped to walk. I heard someone yell "Jackie!" I looked over to my right and there was Roy running to catch up with me. What a glorious sight. I am always so happy to see my husband. *Were those red roses he was carrying? Couldn't be.*

I still get emotional just thinking about the finish, and I can't express exactly what I was feeling as I neared the finish line. It was all so surreal. I realized I had just accomplished something very special and I was extremely proud. I am no longer just an average runner. I had just finished the Boston Marathon. My finish time was 5:15:30. What was left to say? It would take a little time to digest all of this.

I was handed a blanket right away and I wrapped it around my shoulders. I sweat a lot when I run and now I was feeling pretty cold. In fact, I started to shiver. It was now after 4:15 p.m. and I was standing in the shade. The temperature had started to drop the closer I got to Boston, and there was no sun to keep me warm. *Where was my Florida sunshine?*

In every other marathon I have run, the finisher medals were given out just past the finish line. I kept walking and looking for the finisher medals for what felt like forever. Right then I wanted that medal more than I wanted food. I was beginning to think they had given out all of the medals because I was behind most of the finishers. I finally found them and placed my medal very proudly around my neck. I really deserved this one.

Somehow Roy went one way and I went another, but thank goodness we found each other in the family reunion area. He was smiling at me and looked so proud. Roy gave me a hug and kiss and the dozen red roses. They were so beautiful. I asked where he'd bought roses and he just said someplace nearby and not to ask how much he paid for them. He wanted to take some pictures, which I was not in the mood for but I agreed and just asked him to hurry.

The walk to the hotel was only a few blocks but it felt like miles. I was not normally this tired after a marathon. I wanted to take a break and sit on a curb for a few minutes, but I worried I would have too difficult a time getting back up and walking again.

When we got back to the room all I wanted was a yogurt and chocolate milk. Roy was willing to do anything for me and he went downstairs to the snack area. In the meantime, I got out of my running clothes and managed to get into the shower. It was maybe the best shower I'd ever had (I'm sure

I say the same thing after each marathon and long Saturday morning run).

Roy came back with my snacks and both tasted wonderful. He said the snack bar attendant hadn't even charged him when he said the snacks were for his wife who had just finished the marathon. People were so nice our entire trip.

We had plans to go to the after party at Fenway Park, and I'd paid for a second ticket for Roy. But there was so much traffic outside the hotel that it would be difficult to get a cab, and I certainly did not feel like walking. I asked Roy if it would be okay to just order a pizza and have it delivered to the room. He really did not feel like going back to Fenway anyway, especially if we had to walk, so he was very thankful that I'd made the suggestion.

He would have done anything I wanted to do. He kept telling me that this day and this trip were all for me. It was not just "my day," it was "our day." I had finished the Boston Marathon and it was Roy's birthday. As I mentioned earlier, April 18 would turn out once again to be a very special day. The marathon was held on the 18th, Roy's birthday is the 18th, and this was my 18th marathon. Perhaps the time is now for me to become a betting person.

As we stretched out on the bed, we finished off most of the veggie pizza, which was excellent. This was my first meal since breakfast much earlier in the day. It was now 7:30 p.m. and time for bed. What a day. This was one for my running log. It was absolutely worth it all. I was very happy. I told Roy happy birthday one more time and I love you, and was asleep before my head hit the pillow.

The day after the marathon, it was time to go back home. I had slept really well and we were up by our usual 6:00 a.m.

even without a wake-up call. I was a little sore but not too bad. When we went out for breakfast I was excited to wear my marathon shirt, finisher medal, and new jacket. It was time to show off a little; I deserved it.

As we walked through the airport terminal, I saw other people in their marathon shirts or jackets. I wore my jacket proudly. So many people said congratulations. We had a nice flight and it was great to be home. I even managed to get my roses home safely and keep them beautiful for a whole week.

Over the next few days, I thought about the time I spent training to qualify for Boston. The time spent waiting to sign up for the marathon after I ran my qualifying time. The time spent waiting to see if I was accepted to race. The time spent training for the marathon. Now it was all over, except for the memories.

Was it worth it all? Damn right, it was. The entire experience was better than I had ever expected. After all the years of running, racing, and finishing 17 marathons with Boston never ever being a goal, Boston turned out to be a very special surprise. What was the reason for all of this? There must be a reason. I believe everything happens for a reason but this one I couldn't figure out. At least, not that day.

On Thursday I woke up at my usual time, 6:00 a.m. I still couldn't believe it was all over. By now I was feeling really well. I took 10 days off from running. I still stretched, exercised, used hand weights, did some yoga stretches, and walked for an hour each day. The weather was beautiful in Melbourne, so I could also spend time outside and work with my plants.

After the 10 days off, I started running again but just four miles, five days a week. On May 7, I ran a 5K race. I had participated in the Run for the Gecko eight times and had placed in my age group each time. I felt ready to race, and I felt great during the race. I finished in 30:56 and came in First Place in the women's division 65-69. My finish time was a little slower than normal but I didn't mind.

I tried to get back to my normal running and racing schedule, but a few issues had developed.

35

The Year After Boston

When purchasing new running shoes, trust the experts at your local running store.

One thing I was not prepared for after the Boston Marathon was the let-down and sadness that set in. After each of the previous 17 marathons I had always felt great. I would go to work the next day and was never so sore that I could not get out of bed. I might take a week off from running, but then I was right back on the road. I was proud and energized after each accomplishment.

Now I was sad, but not depressed; I still got out of bed each morning at 6:00 a.m. looking forward to my day. I exercised and ran each morning. I took care of our home, the plants outside, and the food shopping and preparation. I had volunteer projects, including a student I mentored at her school on Wednesdays. I sat outside on the porch for a couple of hours most afternoons and read my magazines or a book. I had a good life and very little to complain about.

But still I could not shake this sadness, nor could I explain it. Was it because I'd decided Boston was my last marathon? I don't think so. I had made the same decision several times in the past and felt good about it. Yet, I could not get excited about the new race season coming up, including the Space Coast Half Marathon at the end of November. I was in a funk.

I was happy to get back to my Saturday morning runs on May 28. The temperature and humidity were creeping up once again, but I didn't mind.

In June, I purchased two new pairs of running shoes, a particular brand and style that I had worn and liked years earlier. The ads promised great performance and I just had to have these shoes, even though the experts at Running Zone told me they were not stability shoes. I still thought I would be okay, and the new shoes actually felt good to run in.

On the fourth of July I ran the Firecracker 5K. I finished in 30:58 and placed First in the women's division 65-69. On August 13, I ran the 5K I Run for Pizza, finished in 30:45, and again placed First in my age group. I was noticing a difference in my finish times, running about two minutes slower in a 5K than I had gotten used to expecting of myself. I was sure age had nothing to do with slowing down and that it must be something else.

On August 27, I ran the Running on Island Time 5K in 31:28 and placed number two in the women's 65-69 age division. I was definitely slowing down. This was about the time my left hamstring and right IT band issues were beginning to show up, but this was a Space Coast Runner's series race and I didn't want to miss it.

I normally don't make a big issue out of aches and pains or note in my running log when a pain starts, but I don't remember ever experiencing this kind of pain before. I tried everything I could think of: Epsom salt baths, stretching, massage, and chiropractic adjustments.

I took the first week of September off from running. I was slowing down too much due to the issues with my legs. I continued to work out and walk for an hour each day; I could not stand to just sit around.

September 10 was the Turtle Krawl 5K. This was a fun race near the beach in Brevard County and was well-attended. I put in some miles the days before the race but no further than four miles on the days I ran. My legs were feeling much better, although I was not back 100%.

My left hamstring really bothered me but I was sure I could run a 5K. I got to Mile 1 and my left leg just locked up. I could not run another step. I walked for a few minutes and tried to run again. It was not happening. I walked a few more minutes then tried to run again. Still not happening. I had never in all my years of racing dropped out of a race. I walked the rest of the way to the finish and completed the race in 43:58. I needed to figure this out. My running days could not be over.

36

Hurricane Matthew Comes to Call – Twice!

Make a change if you want different results.

I took two weeks off from running. Roy and I flew to Aruba on September 27 to celebrate our twentieth wedding anniversary. That trip took a little sting out of not running. I did more stretching than anything else, along with short runs on the treadmill and some hand weights. Most of our exercise was walking on the beach.

We were having a great time the first three days, just taking it easy and spending time on the beach. We met many young couples who were there on their honeymoons. Then, we were awakened during the night by very hard rain and winds. Hurricane Matthew, a Category 5, passed about 100 miles off the coast of Aruba. One hundred miles sounds like a long way away, but a Category 5 hurricane can still wreak havoc.

After we got out of bed the next morning we checked out the damage. There was a lot of water covering the outside floors of the resort, and many downed palm trees. Some of the guest rooms were flooded and guests were moved to other rooms. We had to cancel water sports and other activities, but we had a beach to walk on so we were fine and we still had a good time.

Unfortunately, we seemed to bring the hurricane back to Florida with us. Once we knew for sure the hurricane would be close to land, Roy put up the hurricane shutters, then he and some of the other neighbors put up shutters for neighbors who needed help. We live far enough from the beach that we weren't worried about flooding or storm surge, mainly wind damage. We called some friends who live on the beach side and offered our home as a place to stay if they needed to evacuate. The lake behind our house would peak before it was close to our back porch. We didn't think we would have any damage to our house.

Roy and I spent two days bringing in the patio furniture and outdoor plants that were in pots. Anything that could fly needed to be secured. We felt very safe in our house. Matthew passed our way around 7:00 a.m. on Friday morning. After Matthew left us, we went outside to access the damage. Our beautiful yard that I take such good care of was a mess. The grass was almost fully covered with leaves from our two Magnolia trees and neighbor's oak trees. We lost some in-ground plants but not too many. The ones we had left I babied for many months until they looked happy again.

We had no power in our community for three days. We ate as much food from the fridge as we could for a couple of days, then anything left over I threw out, though I hate to waste food. Roy grilled the little bit of meat we had in the freezer and kept it in coolers (though ice was also hard to come by), eating it over the next couple of days. We stayed at our house and waited for the power to come back on, while many of our neighbors checked in to hotels.

We had more damage here in Brevard County than we'd seen in Aruba. A year later most of the damaged boat docks were still not rebuilt or repaired. Roy and I spent another two days taking down the shutters and putting the patio furniture back onto the back porch, along with the plants we'd placed in the garage. I was not running, so I spent several days cleaning and raking the front and back yards. That was good exercise!

On October 3, I tried running again, beginning with two-mile runs and walked the rest of the way home. I stayed with this routine for three days. I had signed up for the Cocoa Beach Half Marathon, which was scheduled for October 23. The previous year I had placed First in my age group and I wanted to run again. I could have willed myself through this one by running and taking lots of walk breaks but I knew better. So, I made the decision to pass and just take care of myself. I hate to sign up for a race and then not run—mostly because I hate to waste money!

I tried again on October 10. I ran three miles each day for two days then took off a few more days. Finally, on October 14, I bought new shoes. I desperately wanted this to be the solution. I thought if it wasn't the shoes creating my problems, my running days just may be over. I had one of the Running Zone experts fit me into the proper stability shoe for me.

In running and in life, begin with one step and make continuous, steady improvements.

I started running three or four miles each day. On Saturday, October 22, I went to the Melbourne Causeway and did my first long run of eight miles. I ran easily for the first four miles and in the second half I took a few walk breaks. I didn't want to push myself; I knew I needed to build back up my mileage slowly.

My mileage continued to improve and so did my legs. The IT band cleared up first, but the left hamstring remained a small issue even though it was getting better. My long runs on Saturdays were back up to 10 miles.

> *If you develop an injury, be very patient until you are pain free. Get back into your normal running routine very slowly.*

In early November we drove down A1A to Key West to attend Meeting of the Minds, the yearly gathering of around four thousand Parrotheads from all over the country (and some from other countries) to "party with a purpose." Roy and I had been taking this trip for several years and I highly recommend it if you like Jimmy Buffett, trop rock, or the Margaritaville lifestyle. Every bar and restaurant has great live music. The only other thing I can tell you is, *what happens in Key West, stays in Key West.*

I had signed up for the Key West Zonta 5K which typically is scheduled when we are down there for the Parrotheads event. I had run this race many times and normally place in my age group. I finished a very disappointing 33:26 and finished number four in my age group. Even though my time was slow, I felt great the entire race and at least now I was running again with very little pain in my hamstring. Was I ever grateful to have the right shoes. I also won a $250 Visa gift card, so that made me feel better.

37

Space Coast Half Marathon
November 27, 2016 – Cocoa, Florida

If you don't quit, you won't stop.

I had signed up once again for the Space Coast Half Marathon. I love this race and this was my tenth year to run. I decided to take it easy even though I was feeling great. I just didn't know if the hamstring would hold up for this distance. I finished in 2:40:00 and did not take any walk breaks. My finish time was much slower as compared to previous years, but I finished pain-free. I finished 7th out of 55 women in my age group, 65-69. I was happy that my body held up. I took a week off from running just to be on the safe side, but I continued to exercise and walk each day. I had no urget to quit running, only a determination to figure out how to keep at it.

I decided that I need to stick with stability running shoes. Wearing the incorrect shoes might have been the reason for my IT band and hamstring issues. From now on I will listen to the experts when I purchase new running shoes!

On December 10, my 68th birthday, I ran the Reindeer Run 5K. I have placed in my age group every year that I have run this race, and this year was no exception. I ran 31:49 and placed

2nd in my age group. My time was slower than I would have liked but I still placed.

We drove to St. Petersburg, Florida, for New Year's Eve. Around 50 of our Parrothead friends were going to the party to close out 2016, a very memorable year for me, and to welcome in the New Year with the wonderful and contagious party-with-a-purpose attitude. Early the next day, January 1, 2017, I started the New Year with a three-mile run.

38

The 30-Year-Old Book

"When anyone tells me I can't do anything, I'm just not listening anymore."
—Florence Griffith Joyner

I had spent months thinking about my experience running the Boston Marathon, and after a few months the sadness started to go away. I think the IT band and hamstring issues took my mind off of being sad as I focused on trying to heal my body.

Every day, vivid memories of qualifying for Boston and running the marathon came to mind. I felt there was a reason for this but could not figure out what it was. Boston had never been on my bucket list, but I still qualified and ran Boston in my late 60s, and the entire process had even seemed easy.

Then, one day it came to me. I felt deep in my soul the reason I was fortunate enough to have had the Boston Marathon experience. There were many lessons in it for me, but certainly a main one was about believing in myself. Negativtiy, fear, and doubts that had been projected onto me during my childhood, and had unfortutnately run the show at times even when I was an adult, had absolutely no place in my life anymore. Not in my mind, not in my body, not in my soul.

Writing a book has been a dream of mine off and on for as long as I can remember. Sometimes I felt it just was not something I could accomplish, but often I felt that I could do it, if only I could ever figure out what to write about. What I realized that day was that I had all of those running logs starting with 1983. I had all of my awards and finisher medals. I had pictures. A voice inside me said, *You have a lot of material*! The research would be so easy, I thought, I don't even need to leave my house to write this book! When it comes right down to it, I had been writing this book for over 30 years.

On July 19, 2016, I started handwriting all of my memories regarding Boston. I wanted to write all of the details while they were fresh in my memory. I gave myself the goal to finish writing my notes by the 2017 Boston Marathon. I sat outside on my patio in the afternoon most days and wrote. I went back through my running log for notes on my training and how I felt.

The morning of the 121st Boston Marathon I finished writing my notes and then sat at my kitchen table to watch the Boston Marathon on TV. I had read stories in *Runner's World* magazine about the elite men and women who would be running that day. Roy had checked the TV listings for me a week before so I didn't need to look for the correct channel. I also had the TV on in the living room so I wouldn't miss a second of this race. I have a difficult time sitting still so I knew I would be up moving around during commercials, maybe doing a little stretching. I had even gotten up to run an hour earlier at 7:00 a.m. so I would be back home for the 8:30 a.m. start.

I opened a new box of tissues, preparing for an emotional morning. I had watched Boston on TV for several years but this year was different. I had an intimate knowledge of this race, now. My own feet had stepped over the starting line and crossed the finish line. I wanted to see how much of the course I remembered. The announcers commented on how steep that first downhill stretch was at the beginning of the race. That I remembered, for sure!

I am not sure of the reason, but I have never studied any marathon course before I start. I think I just like to be surprised. I am going to run the race once I get there, no matter what. I wonder how many people don't sign up for a race if they hear the course is particularly tough? I have heard of runners who study every inch of the course just so they can anticipate everything and feel as prepared as possible. I trust the course will be passable and that I'll figure out how to meet each of its challenges when necessary.

At 8:30 a.m., the physically impaired runners started first. Next were the push-rim participants using a racing wheelchair, first the men and then the women.

At 9:30 a.m. it was time for the women to start. The elite runners were in the front. I recognized a few of them from *Runner's World* magazine and from reading their stories over the years. I admire these women so much!

At almost 10:00 a.m. the elite men were heading to the start, and then they were underway with the first wave of men just behind. It looked like a beautiful morning, just like it had been the previous year. At 10:25 a.m. the second wave of male runners got underway. There was a gentleman in this wave who was running his fiftieth consecutive Boston Marathon. Amazing!

It was now almost 11:15 a.m., my start time last year. There was the small church I remembered near the start. Katherine Switzer was leading Wave 4. She was 70 years old and celebrating her 50-year anniversary of running her first Boston

Marathon. I read her book, *Marathon Woman*, long before I ever considered running Boston, and was very inspired. Ms. Switzer's bib number was 261 and the number would be retired after that year.

The first time I met Ms. Switzer was on November 18, 2009 at Running Zone. That was when I bought the book and she autographed it for me. She wrote a nice note: "Jackie! You've lived a lot of this history, and you know it gives us such joy!" I shared with her how many years I had been running and how many marathons I had completed at the time. She was very nice and interested in everything I shared with her.

I met her again on November 26, 2011, back at Running Zone, and she autographed the book for me again. She wrote: "Jackie – Here you are, 20 pounds lighter and living the running dream! You're inspiring us like crazy! Keep going." I must have told her about my weight loss. At that time, I still did not have plans to qualify for Boston. It would sure be nice for me to be able to tell her I qualified and ran Boston.

As I watched Wave 4 start, I was still thinking about the 11:15 a.m. start time, and how I'd started at 11:15 a.m. the previous year, and had finished around 4:30 p.m. I needed to take another look at my finisher medal to realize I really *had* crossed the finish line at Boston.

When I ran Boston, I'd been surprised at all of the parties along the course, especially in the small towns. As I watched the coverage on TV, I didn't see any of that, just the mass numbers of people cheering along the course. The entire scene was very different when you run the course.

I do remember seeing the Citco sign, but I didn't realize that meant I only had one mile to the finish. A friend of mine from the Space Coast Runners is from Boston and she goes back to

Boston every year to stand near the Citco sign and cheer on the runners. I did not see her when I ran; I was only looking for the finish.

It was now 12:17 p.m. on my watch and Meb Keflezighi had just crossed the finish line. This was his last Boston. My box of tissues was still full at this point, but as I watched Meb being interviewed, I lost it.

Meb broke down and I broke down with him. I could feel his pain as he explained why this was his last Boston Marathon. Meb is a very famous runner. He has a very long list of accomplishments which include: 2009 USA Marathon Champion, 2009 New York City Champion and 2014 Boston Marathon Champion. Although I was not even close to his level, I also struggled with the idea of not running another marathon.

I had received my May issue of *Runner's World* a few days before with Jordan Hasay on the cover. Seeing her live interview after her finish made me tear up again. And again while watching her hug her coach, Alberto Salazar, as they both broke down crying.

Another Boston Marathon had come to an end. More good memories for so many people, especially the runners. I have learned firsthand that you do not need to be an elite runner to have great memories of running the Boston Marathon. Average runners, like me, may have even better memories.

My Boston Marathon medal is a powerful totem to ward off those annoying self-doubts, fears, or negativity…should any of those dare to arise.

39

The End?

Here I sit with my laptop on May 12, 2018, still trying to get this all on paper. I have been trying to come up with a good ending, and then it hit me—my story has not ended! It could go on for years. I am excited about tomorrow and the days after. I still have many miles left in me and races to look forward to.

Back on the day when I put on my first pair of running shoes and ran around the block in Kennesaw, Georgia, I had no idea I would still be running more than 30 years later. I had no idea I would complete 18 marathons. I am not even sure at that time I had even heard of the Boston Marathon.

I had no idea that I would be married for a third time (thank God for this nice surprise). Today I feel I've finally got myself together. It took some time and a lot of work, and running has been a big part of my journey. Running built my confidence and courage. Running gave me something positive to look forward to each day no matter how badly my day was going. At the end of each day I still had my run to look forward to first thing the next morning. If nothing else, my day would start on a positive note.

As I wrote my story I noticed several times over my life when I'd felt like something was missing in my personal life—like there was a hole in my soul. I finally found that missing part and that hole in my soul has finally closed.

Today Roy and I celebrate 23 years since our first date. I think I have lightened up over the past 23 years, thanks to my wonderful husband. He makes me laugh when we first wake up each morning and before falling asleep each night. I no longer feel so tight and angry inside. I feel much more peaceful and this inner peace shows on the outside. Roy is even more supportive of my running today than he was 23 years ago (although he can do without those 5:00 or 5:30 a.m. mornings for long runs or races).

I truly hope my story gives you inspiration. Inspiration to go out and accomplish your own dreams. It might take some time to accomplish your dreams, but never give up. And don't let anyone talk you out of your dreams no matter how impossible or crazy they may seem. You are more in control of your life than you realize. If you never received encouragement as a child, learn to give yourself encouragement as an adult. You can reclaim your childhood dreams and you also can create new ones. Being clear about and connecting with your dreams is a great first step.

> "Your dreams will remain just a dream unless you take small and realistic steps towards achieving them."
>
> —Eileen Anglin

When I look back over the earlier years of my life, there are so many situations I could say that I regret. But, I will not do that, because without them I would not be where I am today. I believe that everything happens for a reason. I believe that, even if only one thing had been different, I would not have met my wonderful husband and certainly would not have run the Boston Marathon. And, believe me, I am loving every minute of my life these days.

You never know when something special will happen to you and change your life forever. Just keep your eyes, ears and heart open. Read inspiring books and listen to people you respect. Find the exercise program that is best suited for you and stick with it for life.

Enjoy your running. Enjoy your day. Enjoy the people you choose to have in your life. Enjoy the life you choose. It really is your choice.

See you on the roads and see you at the races! *Run fast!*

Acknowledgements

I thought writing my book would be difficult, but writing the acknowledgments is a real test of my memory. If I've inadvertently failed to mention you here, please know I appreciate you.

I never mentioned to any one, except my mother when I was in 6th grade, that I wanted to write a book. When my years of running journals revealed to me the essence of the book I wanted to write, I finally told my husband my dream of writing a book. Of course, his reaction was, "Let's buy you a laptop so you can get started." Thank you, my wonderful husband, for your support and encouragement.

First, I would like to thank God for all of the Blessings of family, friends, and excellent health. God gave me this body and the understanding that it is my responsibility to take care of it

I am so blessed to have such a wonderful and interesting family. Each of you are very special to me:

Johnny, Gina, Dakota, Bailey, and Austin. Johnny, my son, to whom I have been so proud to be your mother over the years—thank you for a special daughter-in-law. You two have done such an incredible job with your children. I am very proud of all three. Roy always loved it when they were little and called him "Grandpa Goofy."

I never imagined being a step-parent, but you three really surprised me and for that I am grateful. I am very proud to be your step-mom. You have given me six additional grandchildren, all very special and beautiful.

Brian, Sarah, Dylan, Riley and Cameron

Jeff, Vanessa, Karis, Rhone and Grace

And Nick

Many thanks to Barbara Dee, my publishing partner at Suncoast Digital Press, Inc. Now this is an interesting story to me, and just how things have worked out for me the past 24 years. I had finished writing my book and was looking for an agent. (Seems like publishers will only accept a manuscript from an agent.) Roy and I were at a Parrothead Board Meeting when my friend, Laura, asked how my book was going. I told her I was looking for an agent. (I had e-mailed many agents without a response.) Barbara was sitting across from me and said "I am an agent for non-fiction" and handed me her business card. I almost fell off my chair. This was the first time I had met Barbara and, well, we know how that turned out. Thank you so much.

To my editor, Linda Dessau, Ontario, Canada. I first asked her to critique the book before going through the effort and expense of editing. This was my first experience writing a book and I wanted her expert feedback – go or no go. We also know how that turned out. Thank you so much.

To my photographer, Justin, of Justin Torpy Photography. Your work made my book cover better than I could have imagined.

To Denise, co-owner of Running Zone, for taking the time to contribute the Foreword to my book. I appreciate your time in more ways than one over the past 13 years.

My next door neighbor, Maria. Not even knowing my background, she advised me to make the book personal, to be more open with my readers than I had originally planned. So happy I did. I feel the book took a different turn when the personal was included.

Jimmy Buffett for music that always makes me smile. (Roy and I had a dream-come-true vacation for our 23rd wedding anniversary. We flew to Paris to see Jimmy perform, his concert being on the night of our anniversary. All I can say is "WOW".) Thank you, Jimmy, for adding the fun, the music, the "tropical" to the amazing life we now live.

To all of my past running friends in the Annapolis Striders, Annapolis, Maryland. We had some fun road races, trips and I really enjoyed our Saturday morning long runs. A special thanks to Margie, Mary, and Rita, who helped get me through those long Saturday morning runs on Route 450.

To all of my new friends in the Space Coast Running Club. I never thought I would continue to run past the age of 50, but am so happy I did not give it up.

To the elite women runner's who have inspired me through the years: Miki Gorman, Gayle Barron, Joan Benoit Samuelson, Katherine Switzer, Shalane Flanagan, Des Linden, just to name a few.

To the Race Directors of the 18 marathons I have completed. You know we are not crazy—we are the normal ones.

To all of my past Parrothead friends from the Baltimore Club and Chesapeake Club. I will never forget you. So pleased I have reconnected with a few of you on Facebook.

And to all of my new friends in the Space Coast Parrothead Club. We do have many good times: monthly Phlockings, Friendship Fridays, backyard concerts, community volunteer projects and, of course, Meeting of the Minds in Key West, Florida. I never thought I would be having this much fun at this age. Because of you I just feel younger every day. I don't believe any of us are ready to slow down.

To Denise and Don, co-owners of Running Zone and their staff. I have received the best advise from almost every employee regarding the best running shoes for me. I enjoy running the local races that Running Zone organizes. Running Zone is the best when it comes to organizing races. After all, it was the Space Coast Marathon where I qualified for Boston. Thanks for all you do for runners of all ages and abilities.

To all of the chiropractors in the past whom I went to as a patient, and the ones who employed me. I learned so much about the body and how to take care of it. My special thanks goes to my current chiropractor, Dr. Michelle Munnich. You keep me balanced. You know how much you have helped me over the years. I am forever grateful.

A most heartfelt thank you to my good friends Cindy and Joe who introduced me to my wonderful husband. I just can't find words to express my appreciation to you both. Especially to Cindy, who has been such a special friend for over 24 years. I am so grateful we worked for the same chiropractor in Maryland. You two changed my life and Roy's for the better, forever.

To my most precious gift, my husband, Roy. Oh, my God, what can I say. If I get started with a list of all of the reasons I love you so much and how happy I am I would need to write another book. I love you more deeply as the years go by. I don't remember how I thought my life would turn out but since meeting you it has been full of wonderful surprises. I am so very proud of you. You always make me feel loved, needed and appreciated. You have encouraged me to go for my dreams no matter the cost. Over the years I have tried to give back as much to you as you give to me. I finally feel like a whole person.

Jackie Kellner

Jackie@jackiekellner.com

Lightning Source UK Ltd.
Milton Keynes UK
UKHW020215171221
395765UK00009B/879